Health Policy

Application for Nurses and Other Healthcare Professionals

Demetrius J. Porche, DNS, PhD, APRN, FAANP, FAAN

Dean and Professor
School of Nursing
Louisiana State University Health Sciences Center–New Orleans
New Orleans, Louisiana

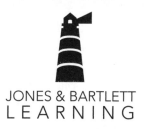

JONES & BARTLETT
LEARNING

World Headquarters
Jones & Bartlett Learning
40 Tall Pine Drive
Sudbury, MA 01776
978-443-5000
info@jblearning.com
www.jblearning.com

Jones & Bartlett Learning
Canada
6339 Ormindale Way
Mississauga, Ontario L5V 1J2
Canada

Jones & Bartlett Learning
International
Barb House, Barb Mews
London W6 7PA
United Kingdom

Jones & Bartlett Learning books and products are available through most bookstores and online booksellers. To contact Jones & Bartlett Learning directly, call 800-832-0034, fax 978-443-8000, or visit our website, www.jblearning.com.

Substantial discounts on bulk quantities of Jones & Bartlett Learning publications are available to corporations, professional associations, and other qualified organizations. For details and specific discount information, contact the special sales department at Jones & Bartlett Learning via the above contact information or send an email to specialsales@jblearning.com.

The author, editor, and publisher have made every effort to provide accurate information. However, they are not responsible for errors, omissions, or for any outcomes related to the use of the contents of this book and take no responsibility for the use of the products and procedures described. Treatments and side effects described in this book may not be applicable to all people; likewise, some people may require a dose or experience a side effect that is not described herein. Drugs and medical devices are discussed that may have limited availability controlled by the Food and Drug Administration (FDA) for use only in a research study or clinical trial. Research, clinical practice, and government regulations often change the accepted standard in this field. When consideration is being given to use of any drug in the clinical setting, the health care provider or reader is responsible for determining FDA status of the drug, reading the package insert, and reviewing prescribing information for the most up-to-date recommendations on dose, precautions, and contraindications, and determining the appropriate usage for the product. This is especially important in the case of drugs that are new or seldom used.

Production Credits
Publisher: Kevin Sullivan
Acquisitions Editor: Amy Sibley
Editorial Assistant: Rachel Shuster
Production Manager: Carolyn F. Rogers
Marketing Manager: Meagan Norlund
V.P., Manufacturing and Inventory Control:
 Therese Connell

Composition and Project Management: DataStream
 Content Solutions, LLC
Cover Design: Kate Ternullo
Cover Image: © Songquan Deng/ShutterStock, Inc.
Printing and Binding: Malloy, Inc.
Cover Printing: Malloy, Inc.

Library of Congress Cataloging-in-Publication Data
Porche, Demetrius James.
 Health policy : application for nurses and other healthcare professionals / Demetrius J. Porche.
  p. ; cm.
 Includes bibliographical references and index.
 ISBN 978-0-7637-8313-6 (pbk.)
 1. Medical policy. 2. Nursing. I. Title.
 [DNLM: 1. Health Policy—United States—Nurses' Instruction. 2. Delivery of Health Care—United States—Nurses' Instruction. WA 540 AA1]
 RA394.P67 2012
 362.1—dc22
                                                            2010039745

6048

Printed in the United States of America
15 14 13 12 11 10 9 8 7 6 5 4 3 2 1

DEDICATION

This book is dedicated to my parents, Hayes James Porche, Jr. and Dianne Lirette Porche; my two sisters, Anastasia Porche Arceneaux and Chelsealea Porche Lovell; my nephews and nieces, Seth Thomas Porche, Sebastian James Porche, Jason Arceneaux, Jasmine Arceneaux, and Madeline Lovell; and my lifetime friend James Arnold Ertl.

TABLE OF CONTENTS

CHAPTER 3—EXECUTIVE BRANCH: FEDERAL GOVERNMENTAL AGENCIES AND APPOINTED BODIES   47

CHAPTER 4—LEGISLATIVE BRANCH: ROLE IN POLICY   61

Chapter 5—Judicial Branch: The Court System

Chapter 6—Public Health Policy

Chapter 7—Policy Formulation and Implementation

CHAPTER 8—POLICY ANALYSIS   131

CHAPTER 9—POLICY RESEARCH, EVALUATION, AND QUALITY IMPROVEMENT   147

CHAPTER 10—POLITICS: THEORY AND PRACTICE   175

CHAPTER 11—POLICY, LAW, AND POLITICS: ETHICAL PERSPECTIVE   217

CHAPTER 12—POLICY INSTITUTES   233

ACKNOWLEDGMENTS

The ability to write a textbook on policy originates from my life experiences and knowledge that has been facilitated by multiple mentors throughout my career. One in particular, who is a lifetime mentor and always available for an immediate mentoring moment, is Dr. Richard Sowell. This book is the result of critical feedback from my graduate students regarding policy courses taught in schools of nursing and schools of public health. To all my students, thanks for challenging and transforming my thinking regarding policy and politics.

PREFACE

The policymaking process is a dynamic and complex process that occurs within a political context. The political context of policymaking is comprised of multiple constituents with varying needs, wants, and desires. In addition, the constituents and policymakers each have varying paradigms that influence and shape their perspective of the societal needs, wants, and desires. The unique paradigm of all individuals involved in the policymaking process also influences the potential solutions and policy alternatives identified during the policy formulation and implementation phases.

Nurses as primary healthcare providers have a wealth of knowledge regarding healthcare systems, clinical practice, academia, and diverse populations that can be maximized with the knowledge of policymaking and politics to influence policy. Nurses and other healthcare professionals have an underutilized potential to impact policymaking processes. This book provides the foundational knowledge regarding the governance structures of our country and the multiple processes that influence and impact policymaking.

Chapter 1 provides an overview of policy. The various types of policy are described along with several policy models. In addition, this chapter introduces the reader to policymakers and policy networks that influence the policymaking process.

Chapter 2 presents the governmental structure in the United States. The US government structure at the federal, state, and local levels is presented. The founding laws and principles for other policymaking decisions are reviewed, such as the Constitution, and the federalism perspective of governmental structure. The branches of government are presented along with an explanation of the federal budgeting process. Government structure at the nonfederal level is discussed with content on state constitutions and city charters.

Chapter 3 presents the various positions and departments within the executive branch of government. The role of the respective executive-level positions and departments in the policymaking process are reviewed.

Chapter 4 reviews the structure of the legislative branch of government. The two chambers of the US legislature are presented along with a discussion of the policy agendas of the two primary political parties in the United States—Democratic and Republican. The legislative process of developing laws is presented, along with the roles and responsibilities of legislative members and staff.

Chapter 5 reviews the role of the judicial system in policymaking, interpretation, and implementation. The structure of the federal, state, and special court systems is presented with a review of the stages of the litigation process. The nurse's role within the judicial system as a legal nurse consultant or expert witness is reviewed.

Chapter 6 focuses on public health policy. Public health policy is directed to preserve the health and welfare of the population. Various types of public health policy measures are presented to ensure the preservation of health in normal and emergency situations.

In Chapter 7, the complex policy formulation and implementation process is reviewed. This chapter presents several policy models that are process oriented and describes the policymaking process from drafting policy proposals to drafting rules and regulations. The nurse's role as a policymaker is presented. This chapter presents the policy implementation process and concludes with policy termination as a means to end current policy or to advance new policy.

Policy analysis models and processes are presented in Chapter 8. This chapter presents the reader with multiple processes that can inform the manner in which they engage in analyzing policy.

The need for and impact of policy is analyzed through the process of policy research and policy evaluation. Chapter 9 presents the research process, research utilization, and evidence-based regulation as possible means to influence policymaking. This chapter presents various policy evaluation models and processes that can be utilized to ensure that policy achieves what was intended. The chapter concludes with quality improvement as a process to further improve policy.

Politics is often a forbidden word in the nursing and other healthcare professions; however, it is a process that every nurse uses daily. Chapter 10 focuses on presenting both the theoretical and practical aspects of politics. This chapter describes many skills that can be used in the political process to influence policy. These skills are presented to provide the nurse with a political toolkit to engage in the policymaking process.

The practice of policymaking and the political activities that influence policy formulation and implementation must occur within an ethical framework. Chapter 11 presents the ethical perspective to ensure that constituents and policymakers engage in an ethical manner consistent with their personal and professional values and accepted ethical codes.

The concluding chapter, Chapter 12, presents the multiple institutes that engage in the policymaking and political process. These policy institutes fund evaluation and research that influence policy or may actively engage in composing positions that influence the thoughts regarding the policy agenda or policy solutions. In addition, many of these institutes and foundations engage in active policy analysis.

The intent of this book is to provide nurses in academia, practice, community settings, and various healthcare systems with an overview of the policymaking process. This book seeks to provide the knowledge necessary to engage in the policymaking process as an influential nurse.

Demetrius James Porche

Policy Overview

Policy and political processes are strategies that nurses and other healthcare professionals can use to implement community- and societal-level change. Policy development and formulation are considered population-based interventions useful in impacting the nation's health. Policy is not random but purpose and goal driven. Policy and politics are interrelated concepts. Policy determines politics and politics determines policy.

Nurses and other healthcare professionals at all educational levels and in all practice settings should strive to become politically knowledgeable and actively participate in policy decision making. Mason, Leavitt, and Chaffee (2006) identified four spheres in which nurses can influence policy: government, workplace, organizations, and community (see **Figure 1-1**). These four spheres can also be applied to other healthcare professionals. These spheres of influence are based on the situational and organizational context in which nurses and healthcare professionals engage in practice. Nurses and some healthcare professionals are employed in government offices and the executive branch. Nurses and healthcare professionals engage in policy development and formulation through their work environment. As professionals, healthcare providers are members of several clinical specialty organizations in addition to organizations of personal interest. As citizens, healthcare professionals are members of communities and in some situations the health-care professional's workplace is encompassed within the community setting. This sphere of influence model emphasizes the healthcare professional's role in impacting policy based on the multiple contextual situations in which these individuals live and practice. In addition, the healthcare professionals are powerful both in numbers and in the intensity of their commitment to impact policy decision making and policy outcomes. Nurses and other health-care professionals are encouraged to capitalize on their collective potential to influence policy.

Policy Defined

An understanding of the word *policy* requires comprehension of multiple definitions and the various manners in which the term is used to convey different meanings. The term *policy* can be used to refer to standing decisions or principles that serve as guidelines for actions. It has also been used to refer to proposals, goals, programs, position statements, or opinions of organizations. Therefore, policy has numerous definitions depending on the context and manner of use. Definitions vary from very simple to complex contextual meanings. The following is a brief summary of multiple definitions of *policy*:

- The principles that govern an action directed toward a given outcome
- A way and means of doing things
- A stated position on an issue
- A plan or course of action selected by any branch of the government or organization
- Authoritative statements, decisions, or guidelines that direct individual behavior toward a specific goal
- Authoritative decisions rendered by any branch of government—legislative, judicial, or executive (Longest, 2005; Mc Lean & Mc Millian, 2010; Titmus, 1974)

The multiple definitions of policy indicate that policy is considered a discipline, an entity or an outcome, and a process for achieving a desired outcome. Therefore, the context in which the term *policy* is used must be considered in order to understand the intended meaning. **Table 1-1** presents other policy-related terms.

Table 1-1   Policy Related Terms

Policy solution	The proposed answer that will resolve the expressed issue or problem.
Private policy	Policy not within the public domain that is typically produced by or governing nongovernmental agencies or organizations.
Policy intention	The expected or anticipated outcome. The policy intention represents what is meant to be achieved by the policy.
Unintended consequences	Sometimes known as policy blowback, these are the unexpected effects that result from the politics surrounding a policy or the development and implementation of a policy.
Policy effect	The measurable impact of a policy which can be intended or unintended.

Policy and Political Theory

Theory attempts to describe, explain, and predict behavior and processes. Theories are made up of concepts and constructs that define the theoretical paradigm that facilitates describing, explaining, and predicting behavior and processes. These concepts are linked together through a theoretical framework that identifies propositional statements. These propositions explain the manner in which the theorist perceives the concepts as related. From a policy and political perspective, characteristics of good theory exhibit a valid representation of reality; economy of scale; testability; heuristic nature; prediction simulation; relevance and usefulness; powerful inferences; reliability through replication; objectivity; veracity; and logical organization (Smith & Larimer, 2009).

Types of Policy

There are multiple types of policy. Policy types are designated based on the intent and focus of the policy. Some policy is not mutually exclusive to one typology. For example, some health policy may also be considered public health policy. In addition to the various definitions of policy, there are different types of policy that further contribute to the meaning of the term. The different types of policy are health, public, public health, social, institutional, organizational, and legal. The type and scope of policy that exists is determined by the governmental structure and political and economic systems. These various types of policy are not always mutually exclusive in their defining characteristics.

Health Policy

Health policy can be generated through governments, institutions, or professional associations. Health policy consists of policy that impacts the health of individuals, families, special populations, or communities. Health policy includes policies that affect the production, provision, and financing of healthcare services. Health policy integrates the definition of health and policy. Health is a concept that is accepted as important to individuals and communities. Some definitions of health are rather simplistic, other definitions define health along a continuum. A simplistic definition of health is the mere absence of disease. Other definitions of health recognize health as existing along a continuum that includes maximal states of positive health and recognizes that an illness or disease process may be present but the individual may experience a positive state of being that is interpreted as "healthy." A generally accepted definition of health at both the national and international level is the World Health Organization's (WHO) health definition. The WHO defines health as a state of complete physical, mental, and social well-being and not merely the absence of disease or infirmity (World Health Organization, 1998).

Health policy builds on this basic definition of health. Health policy, in general terms, is any policy that affects the health of individuals, communities, or society. Health policy is considered a broad type of policy that may include other types of policy such as public policy or public health policy.

Public Policy

Public policy is policy that impacts the general public or citizens. It generally serves the interest of the public. Public policies are authoritative statements generated from the three branches of government—executive, legislative, or judicial—that impact the general public. Defining attributes of public policy are made in the "public's" name, made or initiated by a branch of the government, and interpreted or implemented by the public sector. The definitions of public policy are numerous, without consensus on one definition. The following are some accepted public policy definitions:

- Whatever the government chooses to do or not to do to regulate behavior, organize bureaucracies, distribute benefits, or extract taxes (Dye, 2002)
- The sum of government activities that influences the life of citizens, whether the government acts directly or through other agents (Peters, 1999)
- "A statement by the government of what it intends to do or not to do, such as a law, regulation, ruling, decision, or order, or a combination of these" (Birkland, 2001, p. 132)
- Authoritative decisions made by the three branches of government—executive, legislative, or judicial—that are intended to direct or influence the actions, behaviors, or decisions of others (Longest, 2005)

The definitions of public policy vary by author. However, the definitions of public policy do have common elements or themes. These commonalities focus on governmental influence or regulation and governmental action directed toward individuals or communities.

The World Health Organization further defines what is considered healthy public policy. The WHO (1998) considers healthy public policy as any course of action adopted and pursued (by a government, business, or other organization) that can be anticipated to improve (or has improved) health and reduce inequities in health. Public policy is generally considered a product of some public demand that elicits a government-directed course of action aimed at resolving a problem, or in response to political pressure. The distinctive purposes of public policy are to resolve conflict over scarce resources and provide programs that meet public needs.

Public Health Policy

Public health policy intersects policy that is health related but impacts the general population. It may be defined as "the administrative decisions made by the legislative, executive, or judicial branches of government that define courses of action affecting the health of a population through influencing actions, behaviors, or resources" (Porche, 2003, p. 318). This is in contrast to health policies, which are considered applicable only within specific organizations or institutions, known as organizational or institutional health policy.

Social Policy

Social policy consists of policy that impacts the general welfare of the public. Policy that focuses on meeting the human needs of education, housing, and instrumental social support is typically considered a type of social policy. Some exemplars of social policy areas include:

- Unemployment
- Social security
- Housing
- Education
- Food subsidy programs

Institutional Policy

Institutional policies are policies that are developed or implemented by an institution that affects the respective constituents of the institution. Institutional policies frequently govern the workplace environment. Typical institutional policies consist of policies and procedures outlined in operational manuals.

Organizational Policy

Organizational policies are administrative decisions typically made by a board of directors that outline the decisions, position, or official statements that represent the constituents of the organization. Organizational policies can be in the form of bylaws, policy and procedure manuals, articles of incorporation, resolutions, or position statements.

Legal Policy

Legal policy is generally policy founded upon laws or officially accepted rules promulgated through a legislative or executive governmental process. In addition, legal policy does include case law that is developed through judicial opinions and judgments. Legal policy includes policies that relate to the legal profession. Legal policy includes policy that conforms to the law. Most laws are considered policy but not all policy is considered law or legal policy. For example, institutional and organizational policies may or may not consist of laws or legal policy.

Health, public, public health, social, institutional, organizational, or legal types of policy assume many forms. These various types of policies can be in the form of law, rules or regulations, operational decisions, or judicial decisions. Laws can be enacted at all levels of government. Laws are generally considered free standing legislative enactments that attempt to achieve a predetermined outcome. Laws enacted at the federal or state levels of government are implemented through the formation of rules and regulations by agencies within the executive branch of government. In addition to the formation of rules and regulations, executive branch agencies develop programmatic operational decisions that further implement the intent of the law. These operational decisions can be in the form of policies or procedures. Decisions rendered through the judicial branch can also formulate legal policy. Administrative decisions from the judicial branch are precedent setting in the formation of policy, such as with case law.

Another typology of policy is whether it is substantive or procedural. Substantive policy is policy that significantly changes or alters the current status of events. Procedural policy informs the manner or process in which the policymaking body implements changes.

Policy Intention

Policy is developed and formulated with a specific strategic intention. Two strategies that assist with the implementation of the policy intent are regulation and allocation. A policy with a regulatory intent is designed to prescribe and control the behavior of a particular population. A policy with an allocation intent focuses on providing resources in the form of income, services or goods to ensure implementation of policy to individuals or institutions. Allocation policies can be distributive or redistributive. Distributive policy doles out resources in a planned manner consistent with the policy intent. In contrast, redistributive policy redirects existing resources from a current allocation mechanism to a new direction through a different allocation mechanism.

Policymakers

The policy process engages a variety of different individuals and organizations. Individuals who participate in the development and formulation of policy are referred to as policymakers. Policymakers consist of legislators, executive agency employees, and institutional and organizational administrators and leaders. Individuals who are in, or have privileged access to, the inner circle or upper echelon of Congress, the state legislature, executive agencies, or organizational and institutional leadership are referred to as policy elites. In addition, the policymakers themselves are also referred to as policy elites (Buse, Mays, & Walt, 2005).

Networks

Issue networks consist of individuals or coalitions with an active citizen base that is politically interconnected. These issue networks have specialized policy knowledge especially regarding their issue of interest. Issue networks are considered important to policymakers and the policymaking process. Issue networks generally are aligned with the sentiment of the citizens. In addition, issue networks are a resource that has the ability to apply political power and pressure on policymakers and to generate policy solutions (Smith & Larimer, 2009). Sabatier (2007) refers to policy networks that are similar to what Smith and Larimer describe, and characterizes policy networks as stable patterns of social relations between interdependent constituents that form around a problem or policy. Network management provides the ability to impact these policy networks in the manner desired for collective action.

Network management may be considered a political strategy. Network management consists of controlling and organizing constituents with different goals or preferences in relation to a problem or policy alternative into the same existing relationship network or coordinating divergent efforts within an existing network to impact a specific policy. Network management is also the merging of multiple networks into one network for a common purpose or cause. The effectiveness of network management is dependent upon the number of constituents, the critical mass of constituents needed to exert political power, complexity of existing networks, extent of self-reliance of network, dominance of network, and the degree of conflict of interest between network members and the entire network (Sabatier, 2007).

Policy Decision Making: Influencing Factors

The policy decision-making process is influenced by multiple factors. A general systems model has been used to describe the forces that influence the policy decision-making process. Greipp (2002) identified three major forces that affect policy decision making: consumers, providers, and regulatory bodies. Motivating and inhibiting factors were identified that affect the decision-making process.

Consumers are considered clients, families, and communities. Consumer forces are represented by those who have a perceived need for healthcare services and products. Providers are healthcare professionals who render care to clients, and also scientists or researchers. Providers include family caregivers. The last driving force in health policy decision making is regulatory bodies. Regulatory bodies include governments, legal systems, third-party payers, political action committees, other special interest groups, and ethics and institutional review board committees. These three driving forces interact and influence each other during the health policy decision-making process. The factor with the greatest influence will shape the policy issue and policy adopted (Greipp, 2002).

Motivators and inhibitors are the intervening positive and negative variables that can influence the perspective of consumers, providers, or regulatory bodies. Motivators are the positive variables that influence the decision making in the direction of what is best for the common good. Inhibitors are negative variables that influence the perspective in the direction of self interest rather than public interest (Greipp, 2002).

Agenda Setting

One of the first processes of policymaking, is agenda setting. Many believe that agenda setting is the most critical aspect of policy development and formulation. The word "agenda" indicates that there is some type of prioritization of issues or some listing of issues that is defined as relevant or pertinent. Policymakers must be aware of competing and multiple agendas that influence the public and stakeholder opinion regarding policy. There are typically at least four agendas regarding each issue: media agenda, public agenda, political agenda, and the executive branch/government agenda (Prouty, 2000).

Agenda setting is the process of determining what problems are deserving of policy solutions and resolution at the current time. Kingdon's policy development model proposes the interaction of three policy streams that create a window of opportunity when these respective streams align. These three streams are problem, policy, and political (see Chapter 7). An individual who ensures that the respective problem is brought to the policymaking arena is known as a *policy entrepreneur*. A policy entrepreneur seizes the opportunity within a favorable political climate to bring the policy problem to the forefront of the public agenda for policy development (Kingdon, 1995).

An agenda is a collection of problems, understandings of causes, symbols, solutions, and other elements of public concern that attract the attention of members of the public and/or policymakers. An agenda is also referred to as a coherent set of proposals, each related to the other and forming a series of potential enactments. As stated previously, agenda setting is the process by which problems and potential solutions gain or lose attention and potential for policy action. There are multiple levels of agenda. Each agenda level brings the issue or policy closer to the action potential of policymaking. The agenda levels are agenda universe, systemic agenda, institutional agenda, and decision agenda. The agenda universe represents all the ideas that could potentially be brought up and discussed within a society or political system. Systemic agenda represent the issues that are commonly perceived by members of a political group or community as meriting some public attention and involving matters within their scope of authority or legitimate jurisdiction for action. Institutional agenda is a subset of the broader systemic agenda. The institutional agenda represents the items explicitly being given consideration for action by the policymakers. Lastly, the decision agenda contains those items that are actively on the table for policymaking action by policymakers. **Figure 1-1** presents a model of the policy agenda levels (Kingdon, 1995). The movement of issues through the various levels of an agenda is influenced by multiple variables.

Agenda setting is influenced by interpersonal social and political networks. These networks exert considerable influence on policy agenda setting. This is sometimes referred to as interpersonal agenda setting. Interpersonal agenda setting uses social or political networks to mediate relationships among involved stakeholders and constituents such as policymakers, governmental representatives, elected officials, media, and the general public, to influence the agenda and ultimately policy.

Other driving forces of agenda setting consist of the problem's magnitude, research, political forces, public opinion, and the government's executive official. Problems that are defined and placed on the policy agenda for policy formulation are generally broadly identified by policymakers as important or requiring urgent action to resolve a public health or safety issue. In addition, the perceived magnitude of a problem can be influenced by the amount of

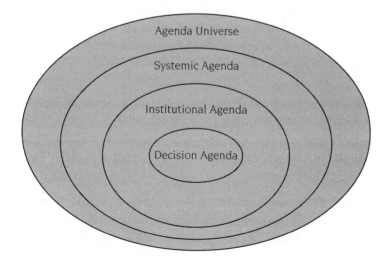

Figure 1-1 Agenda levels model.

public salience and amount of conflict surrounding the respective problem or policy. Problems that have a broad or widespread implication are more likely to be placed on the policy agenda for policy development and formulation. The placement of a problem on the policy agenda is also dependent upon the social and political context of the circumstances surrounding the problem at the given time (Longest, 2005).

A problem represents an unsettled matter that demands a solution or decision. Two general requisites of a *problem* are a perplexing or vexing situation, and an invitation for a solution. A problem is generally considered an area in which there is a discrepancy between what is wanted (desired situation) and what exists (current situation). Sabatier (2007) proposes that problem analysis consists of examining the participants, positions, outcomes, action-outcome linkages, level of control participant's exercise, information available, and the cost and benefits associated with developing a policy to resolve the problem.

Research data provide support for the policy agenda. Research data, such as epidemiological data, outline the determinants of a problem and proposes the impact of an issue, for example through morbidity and mortality statistics. Research determines the extent and nature of a problem, clarifies the associative or related factors, and provides evaluative data regarding potential policy alternative solutions. Research data clarify the problem for placement on the policy agenda. In addition, research presents data that form the baseline foundation for future comparison and measurement of the policy impact and outcomes (Longest, 2005).

Political forces influence the likelihood of a problem being placed on the policy agenda. Problems or policies directly related to a political party's platform are more likely to be placed on their policy agenda. Chapter 10 provides more detail on the influence of politics on policy formulation.

Public opinion's interaction with media creates a cyclic agenda-setting process. The media informs public opinion, and public readership impacts the media's focus on problems or issues of public interest. Each informs the other within the policy agenda setting process. Public opinion can be shared directly with elected officials, through special interest polls, and communicated with the press through letters to the editor.

The governmental elected officer (e.g., president, governor, or mayor) commands the attention of the public and media. These elected officials frequently communicate to the public through the media. During this communication, they are informing the public using the media as a means to prime and frame the problems. These governmental officers have the ability to communicate in the public domain their expected direction for problem resolution and the proposed policy resolution. Formal forums used to communicate these issues are framed as "State of the State" or "State of the Union" speeches. These speeches frequently outline the respective governmental elected officer's policy agenda (Longest, 2005). The manner in which the problems are outlined and policy resolutions are presented frame our thinking regarding the viable policy options and expected outcomes.

Policy Models

A *model* is a description of a complex entity or processes in an understandable manner. A model is sometimes described as a complex program, process, or entity that is replicable within other similar situations. Models are designed to be summative in nature. A model may be composed of a narrative description with an associated figure detailing the relationships between the concepts, variables, or items represented in the model. A policy model is a description of the complex process of developing, implementing, and evaluating the policies and the policymaking processes within a political sphere of influence. Some policy models are presented in the following material and in Chapter 7. These policy models are used to explain the policymaking process but can also be used as a framework to conduct policy analysis (see Chapter 8).

Hall Agenda Setting Model

The Hall Agenda Setting model proposes that an issue or problem emerges on the policy agenda when three criteria are strongly met. These three criteria are legitimacy, feasibility, and support. Legitimacy of an issue or problem is established if the policymaking body believes they have an obligation to engage. Feasibility represents the potential ability to implement the policy solution. Feasibility is dependent upon the availability of necessary resources, such as knowledge, human, fiscal, and physical. Support refers to the amount of public support for the issue or problem (Buse, Mays, & Walt, 2005).

Policy Triangle Model

The policy triangle model is a simplified approach to understanding the policy making process using four inter-related factors. Buse, Mays, and Walt (2005) propose four factors that define the policy triangle as policy context, policy process, policy content, and actors. The policy context consists of the systemic factors that have an impact on the policy solution. Policy context also consists of situational factors (transient conditions that impact policy), structural factors (unchanging elements of society), cultural factors (value and belief systems), and exogenous factors (level of interdependence or level of sovereignty). The policy process is the systematic process of policymaking (problem identification, policy formulation, policy implementation, and policy evaluation). The policy content consists of the policy resolution. Actors are individuals who engage in the policymaking process such as constituents, interest groups, or legislators (Smith & Larimer, 2009).

Politics, Policy, and Values Model

Policymaking is considered a complex, multidimensional, dynamic process that is influenced by the values of those individuals who establish the policy agenda, determine the policy alternatives, define the goals to be achieved by the policy, the implementation methods, and ultimately the manner in which the policy is evaluated. This model asserts that the value framework of everyone involved provides the large context in which decisions are rendered. Politics is the next contextual sphere that is within the espoused value system and also provides a comprehensive context in which the policymaking process occurs. At the core of the model exist the policymaking stages, which are circular and repetitive. These stages consist of agenda, goals, policy alternatives, policy selection, policy implementation, policy evaluation, then cycling back to agenda setting. Politics influences each step of the process (Mason, Leavitt, & Chaffee, 2006).

"Garbage Can" Model

This model proposes that there are policy solutions that have been previously discarded as possible or applicable that remain circulating with the potential policy sphere. These discarded policy solutions might get attached to an identified policy issue or problem (Hanney, Gonzalez-Block, Buxton, &

Kogan, 2003). This discarded policy solution may or may not be appropriate to the problem or issue but gets attached as a viable solution.

Contextual Model

Policy models provide the framework to understand policy and the policy-making process. The contextual policy model proposes at least five contextual dimensions to define the environment which influences policymaking. This contextual model of policy can also facilitate policy analysis. The five contextual dimensions are:

- Complexity and uncertainty of the decision-system environment
- Potential for constituent feedback
- Ability by constituents to control policy formulation
- Stability of constituents and policymakers over time
- Activation of the interested parties

Schneider and Ingram Social Construction Model

The social construction model emphasizes the role of the target population's influence in policymaking processes. Schneider and Ingram (1993) propose that the policymaking process can best be understood by knowing the legislative official's perception of target populations and their respective needs. They further propose that the target population can be categorized as advantaged, contenders, dependents, or deviants. The manner in which the respective target population is seen and categorized will determine the level of influence the respective group has over policymaking. The social construction model perceives target populations along two dimensions, positive or negative, and powerful or powerless. The target populations are perceived in relation to their relative power base and ability to influence policy. For example, children and disabled persons can be categorized as dependent and are viewed very positively but may be perceived as having less power than other groups.

In addition, Schneider and Ingram propose five categories of tools used to influence the policymaking process. These tools are authority, incentive, capacity-building, symbolic and hortatory, and learning (Schneider & Ingram, 1990). Authority tools are statements substantiated by legitimate forms of governmental power that grant permission or prohibit specific actions in certain circumstances. Incentive tools are motivators that influence an individual to engage in volitional behavior to receive the motivator. Capacity-building tools provide needed education, training, or resources to empower individuals to make decisions or engage in activities. Symbolic and hortatory tools use the individual's internal motivation as a catalyst for action based on their beliefs and values. Learning tools use needs assessment data to identify the informational needs and inform the needed policy.

Political Influence Model

Political influence represents the ability of an individual or group to impact the policy agenda and policy development and formulation process. The political influence model proposes that nurses have the ability to significantly influence policy development, formulation, and implementation within four spheres. The four spheres of influence are government, workplace, organizations, and community. A nurse's active engagement in these environments provides the nurse with an opportunity to advocate for specific policy agendas and influence policy development and formulation from a nursing perspective. Other healthcare professionals as well as nurses can engage in political influence within these four spheres. **Figure 1-2** presents visual representation of the political influence model.

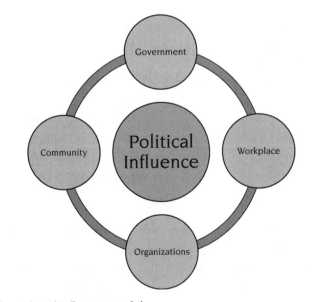

Figure 1-2   Political influence model.

6 Ps Model

The 6 Ps policy model provides a simplistic framework from which to understand the multiplicative factors that influence policy development. The 6 Ps policy model consists of policy, process, players, politics, press, and public polls. **Figure 1-3** depicts the aspects of the 6 Ps policy model.

Problem-Centered Public Policymaking Process Model

The problem-centered public policymaking process model presents a complex, dynamic, nonlinear, cyclical, and iterative process that can be used to understand policymaking and to analyze policy. The model is considered to

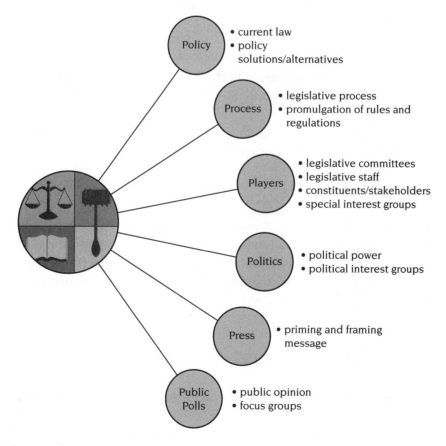

Figure 1-3   6 Ps policy model.

revolve around a central core element, the problem. A premise of the model is that problem recognition and correct identification of the "real" problem are necessary conditions for the policy-making process. This model considers the major players in the policymaking process to consist of legislators, members of the executive branch, and members of interest groups. This model recognizes that policymaking and policy analysis are two separate processes; however, these activities may occur concurrently as a means to formulate or modify policy. The six phases of the problem-centered public policy-making process are:

- Agenda setting—the initial and crucial phase that uses Kingdon's three streams—problems, policy, and politics to determine the readiness of the window of opportunity to develop policy
- Policy formulation—identifying policy alternatives and developing or formulating the selected policy alternative
- Policy adoption—selection of the policy
- Policy implementation—mobilization of the physical, human, and fiscal resources to carry out the intended policy
- Policy assessment—determining the extent to which the policy implementation is in alignment with the intention, statutory requirements, and expected objectives
- Policy modification—using the policy assessment to modify, maintain, or eliminate the implemented policy (Dunn, 2009)

Punctuated Equilibrium (PE) Model

Punctuated equilibrium describes the process of achieving policy change. This model proposes that policymaking occurs through incremental changes that occur over an extended period of time. These extended periods of incremental policy changes are followed by brief periods of major or transformational policy change (Sabatier, 2007).

Policy Cycle–Process

The formation and implementation of policy experiences revision as findings from policy analysis, policy evaluation, and policy research informs policymakers of needed changes in the current policy. This process is referred to as the policy cycle. The policy cycle is composed of 10 components that are cyclic:

issue raising, agenda setting, policy drafting, public support building, policy-maker support building, policy development and formulation, policy passage, policy implementation, policy evaluation, and policy revision. **Figure 1-4** depicts the policy cycle. *Policy* consists of the current laws and policies that are competitive and similar along with all potential policy solutions and alternatives. *Process* includes the legislative processes required to evolve from policy idea to draft policy. Depending on the level of policy development—federal, state, or within an executive agency—the policy process may include the promulgation of rules and regulations in accordance with administrative law and procedures. Players include all individuals and groups that have a vested interest in the problem or policy resolution. Politics consists of the processes utilized to influence the public, legislators, or other stakeholders regarding the

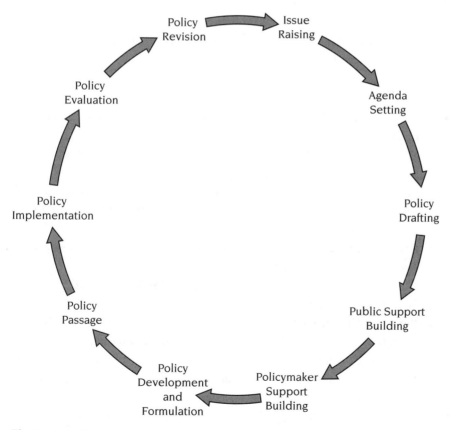

Figure 1-4 Policy cycle.

desired course of policy action. Press represents the media message regarding the problem or policy resolution. Lastly, public polls provide a real-time assessment of public opinion regarding the proposed policy (Hall-Long, 2009).

Policy on Policy

A policy on policy is a guidance document regarding several aspects of the policymaking process. Policy on policy implies that a policy is generated to outline the terminology used in the policymaking process, the manner in which policies are made, the policy approval process, the time interval for reviewing policies for modification and change, and frequently outlines the policy model for the governmental body, organization, or institution.

Summary Points

- Policy and political processes are strategies that nurses and other healthcare professionals can use to implement community- and societal-level change.
- Four spheres in which nurses and other healthcare professionals can influence policy are government, workplace, organizations, and community.
- The term *policy* has been used to refer to proposals, goals, programs, position statements, or opinions of organizations.
- The multiple definitions of policy indicate that policy is considered a discipline, an entity, or an outcome, and a process of achieving a desired outcome.
- The different types of policy are health, public, public health, social, institutional, organizational, and legal.
- Health policy consists of policy that impacts the health of individuals, families, special populations, or communities.
- Public policies are authoritative statements generated from the three branches of government—executive, legislative, or judicial—that impact the general public.
- Public health policy intersects policy that is health related but impacts the general population.
- Social policy consists of policy that impacts the general welfare of the public.

- Institutional policies are policies that are developed or implemented by an institution that affects the respective constituents of the institution.
- Organizational policies are administrative decisions typically made by a board of directors that outlines the decisions, position, or official statements that represent the constituents of the organization.
- Legal policy is generally policy that is founded upon laws or officially accepted rules promulgated through a legislative or executive governmental process.
- Most laws are considered policy but not all policy is considered law or legal policy.
- A policy with an allocation intent focuses on providing resources in the form of income, services, or goods to ensure implementation of policy to individuals or institutions.
- Distributive policies dole out resources in a planned manner consistent with the policy intent.
- Issue networks consist of individuals or coalitions with an active citizen base that is politically interconnected.
- Network management consists of controlling and organizing constituents with different goals or preferences in relation to a problem or policy alternative into the same existing relationship network or coordinating divergent efforts within an existing network to impact a specific policy.
- Individuals who are in, or have privileged access to, the inner circle or upper echelon of Congress, the state legislature, executive agencies, or organizational and institutional leadership are referred to as policy elites.
- Three major forces that affect policy decision making are consumers, providers, and regulatory bodies.
- There are typically at least four agendas regarding each issue: media agenda, public agenda, political agenda, and the executive branch/government agenda.
- Agenda setting is the process of determining what problems are deserving of policy solutions and resolution at the current time.
- Kingdon's policy development model proposes the interaction of three policy streams that create a window of opportunity when these respective streams align. These three streams are problems, policy, and politics.

- Agenda setting is influenced by interpersonal social and political networks.
- Policymaking is considered a complex, multidimensional, dynamic process that is influenced by the values of those individuals who establish the policy agenda, determine the policy alternatives, define the goals to be achieved by the policy, the implementation methods, and ultimately the manner in which the policy is evaluated.
- The six phases of the problem-centered public policy-making process are: agenda setting, policy formulation, policy adoption, policy implementation, policy assessment, and policy modification.
- The policy cycle is composed of 10 components that are cyclic: issue raising, agenda setting, policy drafting, public support building, policymaker support building, policy development and formulation, policy passage, policy implementation, policy evaluation, and policy revision.
- Policy on policy is a guidance document to the entire policymaking process for a governmental body or organization.

References

Birkland, T. (2001). *An introduction to the policy process: Theories, concepts, and models of public policy making.* Armonk, NY: M. E. Sharpe.

Bobrow, D., & Dryzek, J. (1987). *Policy analysis by design.* Pittsburgh, PA: University of Pittsburgh Press.

Buse, K., Mays, N., & Walt, G. (2005). *Making health policy.* Berkshire, UK: Open University Press.

Dunn, W. (2009). *Public policy analysis: An introduction* (4th ed.). Englewood Cliffs, NJ: Prentice Hall.

Dye, T. (2010). *Understanding public policy* (13th ed.). Upper Saddle River, NJ: Prentice Hall.

Greipp, M. (2002). Forces driving health care policy decisions. *Policy, Politics and Nursing,* 3(1), 35–42.

Hall-Long, B. (2009). Nursing and public policy: A tool for excellence in education, practice, and research. *Nursing Outlook,* 57, 78–83.

Hanney, S., Gonzalez-Block, M., Buxton, M., & Kogan, M. (2003). The utilization of health research in policy-making: Concepts, examples and methods of assessment. *Health Research Policy and Systems,* 1(2), 1–28.

Kingdon, J. (1995). *Agendas, alternatives, and public policies* (2nd ed.). New York, NY: Longman.

Longest, B. (2005). *Health policymaking in the United States* (4th ed.). Washington, DC: Association of University Programs in Health Administration.

Mason, D., Leavitt, J., & Chaffee, M. (2006). *Policy and politics in nursing and health care* (5th ed.). St. Louis, MO: Saunders.

Porche, D. (2003). *Public & community health nursing practice: A population-based approach.* Thousand Oaks, CA: Sage.

McLean, I., & McMillan, A. (2010). *The concise Oxford dictionary of politics* (3rd ed.). Oxford, England: Oxford University Press.

Peters, B. G. (1999). *American public policy: Promise and performance.* Chatham, NJ: Chatham House Publishers.

Prouty, J. (2000). *Agenda setting function of Maxwell McCombs & Donald Shaw.* Retrieved from http://oak.cats.ohiou.edu/~jp340497/agsapp.htm

Sabatier, P. (2007). *Theories of the policy process* (2nd ed.). Boulder, CO: Westview Press.

Schneider, A., & Ingram, H. (1993). Social construction of target populations: Implications for politics and policy. *American Political Science Review, 87*(2), 334–347.

Schneider, A., & Ingram, H. (1990). Behavioral assumptions of policy tools. *Journal of Politics, 52*(2), 510–529.

Smith, K., & Larimer, C. (2009). *The public policy theory primer.* Boulder, CO: Westview Press.

Titmus, R. (1974). *Social policy: An introduction.* New York, NY: Pantheon.

World Health Organization. (1988). *Adelaide recommendations on healthy public policy.* Retrieved from http://www.who.int/hpr/NPH/docs/AdelaideRecommendations.pdf

World Health Organization. (1998). *Health promotion glossary.* Retrieved from http://www.who.int/hpr/NPH/docs/hp_glossary_en.pdf

Governmental Structure

G overnment is an entity, organization, or institution that provides the structure of rule within a defined country or nation. Government is also considered the act or process of governing, especially the development, implementation, evaluation of public policy in a political unit. The purposes of government are multi faceted. The government provides the political and organizational structure to rule an entity (country or nation); protects the interest of the state or sovereignty; develops policies; protects the interests of individuals; provides peace and stability; provides services; and promotes the general welfare of the citizens.

Governmental Structure

The United States Constitution forms the legal basis of the United States legal system. The three primary functions of the US Constitution are to allocate power between the federal government and the states (federalism), divide power among the three branches of government (separation of power), and limit the amount of government power (protection of individual liberties). **Figure 2-1** presents the branches of the US government. **Figure 2-2** shows a comprehensive representation of the government structure (Longest, 2005).

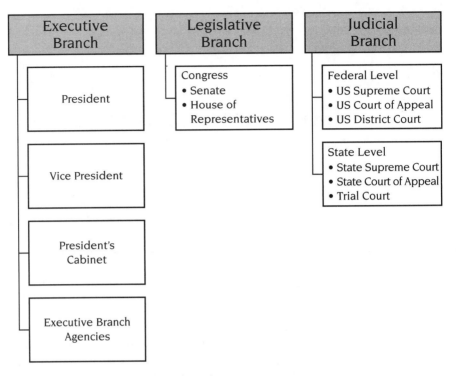

Figure 2-1 United States branches of government structure.

Federal

The federal government of the United States is centered in Washington, DC. The federal government consists of 10 regional offices. **Table 2-1** outlines the states included within each of those regions. At the federal level, the government is composed of the executive, legislative, and judicial branches. These branches are briefly described in the following text, and respectively in Chapters 3, 4, and 5. This federal government structure forms the basis of our system of federalism in the United States.

State

The state governments are organized and structured under state constitutions. The state constitutions are similar to the federal constitution. In a federalist system, each state government mirrors the federal government structure

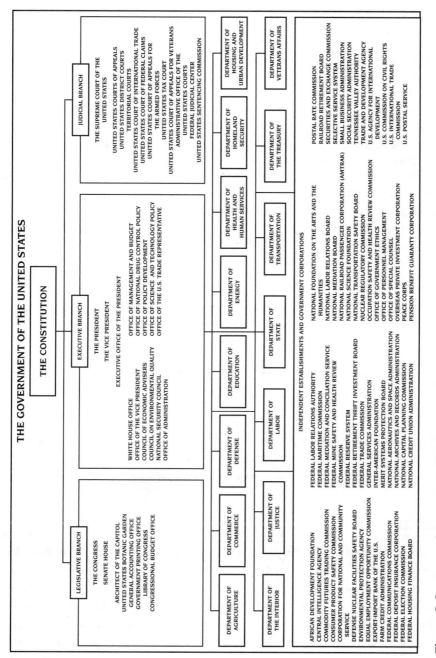

Figure 2-2 Comprehensive United States government structure.

Table 2-1   United States Federal Regions

Region 1
- Connecticut
- Maine
- Massachusetts
- New Hampshire
- Rhode Island
- Vermont

Region 2
- New York
- New Jersey
- Puerto Rico
- Virgin Islands

Region 3
- Delaware
- Maryland
- Pennsylvania
- Virginia
- West Virginia
- District of Columbia

Region 4
- Alabama
- Florida
- Georgia
- Kentucky
- Mississippi
- North Carolina
- South Carolina
- Tennessee

Region 5
- Illinois
- Indiana
- Minnesota
- Ohio
- Wisconsin

Region 6
- Arkansas
- Louisiana
- New Mexico
- Oklahoma
- Texas

Region 7
- Iowa
- Kansas
- Missouri
- Nebraska

Region 8
- Colorado
- Montana
- North Dakota
- South Dakota
- Utah
- Wyoming

Region 9
- Arizona
- California
- Hawaii
- Nevada

Region 10
- Alaska
- Oregon
- Washington
- Idaho

with three branches of government to ensure state-level distribution of power. Again, these branches are executive, legislative, and judicial. State-level laws or policies must not conflict with federal laws or policies.

Local

A state constitution outlines the local governmental structure for the respective state. The local government structure can consists of parishes, counties, cities, and villages. Local governments usually have a governance structure that is parallel to the federal and state government structure. A mayor typically leads the executive branch, which is composed of an elected city council or board. The function of government at the local level is described through either a city charter or city constitution. Laws or policies at the local level must not conflict with either state or federal laws or policies.

Table 2-2   United States Constitution Preamble

"We the People of the United States, in Order to form a more perfect Union, establish Justice, insure domestic Tranquility, provide for the common defence, promote the general Welfare, and secure the Blessings of Liberty to ourselves and our Posterity, do ordain and establish this Constitution for the United States of America."

United States Constitution

The Constitution of the United States is the supreme law of the land. It is the legal reference for the highest judicial decisions in the United States made by the Supreme Court. The Constitution serves as the foundation of, and provides the legal structure for the United States government. It defines the structure, power, and responsibility of the branches of government, and serves as a model document for state constitutions and city charters.

The Constitution consists of a preamble, seven original articles, and twenty-seven amendments. **Table 2-2** presents the preamble. The seven original articles provide the legal foundation for legislative power, executive power, judicial power, state powers and limits, amendment ratification methods, and ratification process of the Constitution itself. Of the 27 amendments, the first 10 represent what is known as the United States Bill of Rights, shown in **Table 2-3**.

Table 2-3   Bill of Rights of the US Constitution

1. Congress shall make no law respecting an establishment of religion, or prohibiting the free exercise thereof; or abridging the freedom of speech, or of the press; or the right of the people to peaceably assemble, and to petition the Government for a redress of grievances.

2. A well regulated Militia, being necessary to the security of a free State, the right of the people to keep and bear Arms, shall not be infringed.

3. No Soldier shall, in time of peace, be quartered in any house, without the consent of the Owner, nor in time of war, but in a manner to be prescribed by law.

(continues)

Table 2-3   Bill of Rights of the US Constitution (*continued*)

4. The right of the people to be secure in their persons, houses, papers, and effects, against unreasonable searches and seizures, shall not be violated, and no warrants shall issue, but upon probable cause, supported by Oath or affirmation, and particularly describing the place to be searched, and the persons or things to be seized.

5. No person shall be held to answer for a capital, or otherwise infamous crime, unless on a presentment or indictment of a Grand Jury, except in cases arising in the land or naval forces, or in the Militia, when in actual service in time of War or public danger; nor shall any person be subject for the same offence to be twice put in jeopardy of life or limb; nor shall be compelled in any criminal case to be a witness against himself, nor be deprived of life, liberty, or property without due process of law, nor shall private property be taken for public use, without just compensation.

6. In all criminal prosecutions, the accused shall enjoy the right to a speedy and public trial, by an impartial jury of the State and district wherein the crime shall have been committed, which district shall have been previously ascertained by law, and to be informed of the nature and cause of the accusation; to be confronted with the witness against him; to have compulsory process for obtaining witnesses in his favor, and to have the Assistance of Counsel for his defense.

7. In suits at common law, where the value in controversy shall exceed twenty dollars, the right of trial by a jury shall be preserved, and no fact tried by a jury, shall be otherwise reexamined in any Court of the United States, than according to the rules of the common law.

8. Excessive bail shall not be required, nor excessive fines imposed, nor cruel and unusual punishments inflicted.

9. The enumeration in the Constitution, of certain rights, shall not be construed to deny or disparage others retained by the people.

10. The powers not delegated to the United States by the Constitution, nor prohibited by it to the States, are reserved to the States respectively, or to the people

Federalism

Federalism separates the legal scope of authority into two governmental tiers, federal and state. Federalism grants the federal government limited authority but allows the state governments plenary powers to protect the public. The chief powers for public health purposes are the powers to tax, to spend, and to regulate interstate commerce (Gostin, 2008). In addition to delegated powers, states maintain the powers that they had prior to the ratification of the US Constitution. The "reserved powers" doctrine holds that states can exercise all powers inherent in government to protect the public through the formation of policies and political structures (Gostin, 2008; Grad, 2004).

Federalism is a government system that provides for shared sovereignty among multiple levels of government in which the national government retains supremacy. There are three essential characteristics that must be present under a federalism structure of governance: (1) There must be a provision for multiple levels of government to act simultaneously on the same territory or on the same citizens. (2) Each of the respective levels of government must have its own sphere of authority and power, which may overlap with the other levels of government. (3) In accordance with the US Constitution, federal law is supreme over state law. Likewise, most state constitutions provide that state law is supreme over local laws and policies (Mueller, 2001).

In addition to being considered a government system, federalism is also considered a political system with a division of political units at the national, state, and local levels. The central purpose of federalism is to ensure protection against tyranny, encourage policy diversity, manage conflict between governmental levels, disperse power, and ensure representation of the people in a democracy. The US Constitution provides for a federalist system; however, it provides protection only for national and state governments. Local governments have delegated powers generally derived from the state constitution. The federalism perspective has changed over time. **Table 2-4** presents the federalist perspective over time in the United States. The perspective can be used in policy analysis to examine the context in which national, state or local policy was developed.

The structure under federalism sets up a hierarchy of powers. In a federalist structure that has a national and state level government, the federal government has preemption over state or local laws. This is permitted through the national supremacy clause in the US Constitution. There are different types of preemption. *Total preemption* exists when the federal government assumes all powers over state laws. *Partial preemption* exists when a policy of the same or similar topic exists at the national and state level. In this situation, partial preemption permits state laws concerning the policy to be valid as long

Table 2-4   Federalism Context in the United States for Policy Analysis

Pre-Federalism Period: 1775 to 1789

- This period of time was marked by the establishment of a national government under the Articles of Confederation.
- A new Constitution was drafted and adopted that formed the federal system of government.
  - ○ 1776—Declaration of Independence
  - ○ 1777—Drafted Articles of Confederation
  - ○ 1781—Articles of Confederation approved by states
  - ○ 1786—Articles of Confederation reconsidered
  - ○ 1787—New Constitution drafted

Dual Federalism Period: 1789 to 1865

- Dual federalism is established with national and state governments as equal partners with distinct scope of authority.
- Period is marked by tensions between the national and state governments.
  - ○ 1789—Constitution approved by States
  - ○ 1789 to 1801—Period known as the Federalist Period—Leaders such as George Washington, Alexander Hamilton, and John Adams promoted the establishment of the federal government.
  - ○ 1791—Ten Amendments added to the Constitution as the Bill of Rights. Congress also established the Bank of the United States.
  - ○ 1798—Doctrine of Nullification passed to permit states to suspend federal laws within its boundaries that were determined unconstitutional.
  - ○ 1815—States' Rights Doctrine urged states to protect citizens against acts of Congress that were not Constitutional.
  - ○ 1819—Doctrine of Implied Powers—Permitted federal government to pass laws that were determined to be "necessary and proper" to carry out Constitutional duties.
  - ○ 1820s to 1830s—States clash over tariffs
  - ○ 1824—Federal regulation of interstate commerce
  - ○ 1842—Testing of Constitution's supremacy clause and States' Rights Doctrine
  - ○ 1850—Fugitive Slave Act and prelude to Civil War
  - ○ 1860—Civil War
  - ○ 1862—Morrill Act—Provided land grants to states to support the expansion of higher education public institutions.

Dual Federalism Period: 1865 to 1901

- Increasing presence of national government in areas traditionally in the purview of the states

(continues)

Table 2-4   Federalism Context in the United States for Policy Analysis (*continued*)

- ○ 1868—Due process and equal protection clauses of the Constitution—Fourteenth amendment added which proposes due process and equal protection clauses. These clauses strengthened the federal government's judicial powers
- ○ 1873 – Doctrine of States' Rights revived—Ensured that state and national citizenship were distinct entities, restored some state powers.
- ○ 1887—Interstate Commerce Commission Act strengthened Congress' role in regulation.
- ○ 1890—Sherman Anti-trust Act—Permitted Congress to control the formation of monopolies.
- ○ 1896—Civil rights' Separate But Equal doctrine—Permitted segregation as long as accommodations were equal. This doctrine was overturned in 1954.

Cooperative Federalism Period: 1901 to 1960

- This era was marked by greater cooperation by multiple levels of government
  - ○ 1910—New Nationalism—Sought to expand the powers of the national government
  - ○ 1913—Sixteenth amendment—Authorizes the federal income tax system and develops "grants-in-aid system."
  - ○ 1933 to 1938—Period of New Deal—Expanded role of government in domestic affairs to include economic and social policy. This was an attempt to impact the economic situation.
  - ○ 1944—McCarran Act—Delegates regulation of banking and insurance to the states
  - ○ 1954—Civil rights and states' rights reconsidered—The 14th Amendment of the US Constitution was used to establish due process and equal protection with a final determination that segregated schools were inherently unequal.

Creative Federalism Period: 1960 to 1968

- The era of the Great Society which further shifted powers to the national government level through the expansion of grant-in-aid programs. Grant-in-aid program regulations were used as a mechanism to induce control over state-level policy. A large number of grants were provided by the federal government during this period.

(continues)

Table 2-4 **Federalism Context in the United States for Policy Analysis**
(*continued*)

Contemporary Federalism Period: 1970 to 1997

- This era experienced an increase in unfunded federal mandates and continual disputes over the federal government systems' amount of regulation.
- Concerns emerged about duplication of services, fragmentation, overlap, and confusion of federal and state responsibilities.

New Federalism: 1970s to 2001

- This period focused on reducing national control over grant programs.
- Decentralization of national programs with revenue sharing
  - ○ 1995 to 1997—Formation of the "Contract with America" and Health Insurance Portability and Accountability Act
  - ○ 1993 to 2001—Presidency of Bill Clinton sought to end the era of government and focus on development and reformation of social programs such as health care, education, and environment.

21st Century Federalism

- 2001 to 2009 – President George W. Bush promoted a federalist centralization of power at the level of the federal government and executive branch. Federalism was depreciated during this period.
- 2009 to Present—President Barack Obama proposes to return the country back to the core principles of federalism. President Obama's roots in community organizing and empowerment proposes a potential paradigm that will support an agenda of shared power and collaboration at multiple levels of government that extends to individual empowerment.

as the state law does not conflict with the federal law. The standard partial preemption permits state laws or regulatory agencies to regulate activities in a field regulated by the federal government as long as the state regulatory policy standards are at least as stringent as the federal policy standards. In contrast to preemption, a federalism structure permits federal mandates. Federal mandates are direct orders or regulations to the state government that require the conduct of specific state activities generally through the enactment of federal laws. If fiscal resources are not allocated to the states for the implementation of these federal mandates or to assist with offsetting the cost of implementation, it is considered an unfunded federal mandate. Some examples of unfunded federal mandates are the Age Discrimination Act, Safe Drinking Water Act, and Americans with Disabilities Act.

The federalist structure is deeply rooted in our American governance structure. The federalism framework of governance structure provides the basic framework that guides the development of organizational or institutional structures, delineation of authority and accountability, and policy processes.

The federalism perspective has changed over time in the United States. The Federalist perspective should be considered as one engages in the policy analysis process. The Federalist perspective provides the context within which policy was developed within the respective time period.

Under the federalist separation of the government into federal and state hierarchies, states are delegated police power. Police power provides the legal authority to ensure the health, safety, and welfare of society. In addition, states are granted parens patriae (patriarchal power) and taxation power.

Police Power

Police was the original term used to describe the powers that permitted the sovereign government the right to control its citizens. The purpose of this was to promote the general health, safety, comfort, morals, and prosperity of the public (Gostin, 2008). The three underlying principles of police power are to promote the greater public good, permit the restriction of private interest to promote public good, and permit pervasiveness of state powers.

Parens Patriae Power

Parens patriae means "parent of the country." Parens patriae power provides the state with inherent power through sovereignty to safeguard citizens of the state. This power basis provides states the legal authority to protect the interests of minors and incompetent persons: States may make decisions on behalf of individuals who are incapable of making decisions for themselves. Parens patriae allows states to assert their own general interest regarding communal health, safety, comfort, and welfare (Gostin, 2008).

Taxation Power

Taxation is a power that regulates individual private behaviors through economic penalties. The power to tax is frequently referred to as the power to govern people's individual behaviors (Gostin, 2008).

Centralism

In contrast to federalism, in which sovereignty is shared, centralism concentrates sovereignty within one governmental structure. Centralism is based on a federal parliament. In this parliamentary structure, the federal parliament has a general power to make laws for the peace, order and good government within the respective country.

Centralism can also be referred to the concentration of power to formulate policy within an organization at one level. From a political perspective, the term centralism is used to denote centrism. Centrism is the political positioning between conservatism and liberalism (Mueller, 2001).

Branches of Government

Governmental power and authority at the national level is separated among the three governmental branches—executive, judicial, and legislative. Executive power is vested in the president of the United States, judicial power is vested in the United States Supreme Court, and legislative power is vested in the United States Congress. Governmental power and authority at the state level maintains a similar governmental structure that separates delegated state powers within the state among three governmental branches.

Executive

The executive branch executes the law through policy enforcement. The executive branch also proposes law to the legislature, issues and enforces regulations, and approves or vetoes proposed legislation. The major components of the executive branch are the Executive Office of the President (EOP), presidential cabinet, and cabinet departments. These are presented in Chapter 3.

Legislative

Congress has three powers that provide the foundation for its influence in the policy process. These three powers are: the power to make all laws, the power to tax, and the power to spend. The legislative branch is composed of two chambers—the Senate and the House of Representatives. Legislative members are frequently referred to as congressional officers or members of Congress. The Senate has 100 seats, representing two members from each state. Senators are elected for six-year terms. The House of Representatives currently has 435 seats in which representation is based on the respective state's population size. This allocation is reviewed every 10 years based on results of the national decennial census. Representatives are elected for two-year terms. Each congressional officer is assigned to one or more committees in the respective chamber. Chapter 4 provides more information on the legislative branch.

Judicial

The judicial branch is the final interpreter of Constitutional and federal statutory law, preserves individual rights and Constitutional structure, and develops a body of case law for precedence. Chapter 5 presents information on the judicial branch of government.

Federal Budget Process

The federal budget process is a collaborative effort between the executive and legislative branch of government. The president, as the official leader of the executive branch of government, sets the national spending agenda, outlined in what is known as the presidential budget. The legislative branch of government evaluates the budget and allocates spending. The federal budget fiscal year extends from October 1 through September 30. The federal budgeting process begins each year in early February. The Senate and House of Representatives compose budget resolutions for their respective chambers. The federal budget should be passed during March through each respective chamber. Once the budget is passed, a conference committee, with representation from each chamber, convenes to propose a single budget resolution with an anticipated passage date of April 15. **Table 2-5** presents the budget process timeline.

After the budget resolution is passed, budget reconciliation legislation is composed along with appropriation bills. The reconciliation bill is legislation that reconciles the governmental revenue (primarily from taxation) with the

Table 2-5   Budgeting Process Timeline

First Monday in February
Deadline for submission of president's budget.

February 15
Deadline for submission of Congressional Budget Office (CBO) report on
   projected spending for the forthcoming fiscal year
CBO examines president's budget
CBO examines economic impact of president's budget

Six weeks after the president's submission
Deadlines for the congressional standing committees to submit comments
   regarding the president's budget to the House and Senate budget committees

March
House and Senate budget committees develop separate budget resolutions
House Budget Committee reports in March, and the full House votes on the
   budget resolution about a week later.

April 1
Deadline for Senate Budget Committee to report budget resolution
Full Senate expected to act on its budget resolution about a week later.

April 1–15
House and Senate conference committees develop a conference report on a
   budget resolution.
Each respective chamber votes on the resolution from the conference committee.

April 15
Congress expected to complete action on the concurrent budget resolution,
   generally referred to as the budget resolution, or the budget.

April 15–May
Authorizing committees develop reconciliation legislation
Reconciliation legislation reported to budget committees of each respective
   chamber
Budget committee acts on this proposed legislation (reconciliation legislation) and
   sends it to the respective chamber floor
Each respective congressional chamber acts on this reconciliation legislation
After passage, a House and Senate conference committee develops a report for
   final authorizing legislation.

May 15
Target date for the House to consider annual appropriations bills

June 10
House Appropriations Committee reports out, approves, and sends to the floor
   the final annual appropriations bill for a vote.

(continues)

Table 2-5   Budgeting Process Timeline (*continued*)

June 15
Congressional target date to complete action on reconciliation legislation

June 30
Target date for the House to complete action on annual House appropriations bills

July 1-September 30
Senate completes action on Senate appropriations bills
House and Senate conference committees complete action on appropriations
    conference reports and bring them to the floors their respective chambers.

September 30
Congressional fiscal year ends

October 1
New fiscal year begins

---

amount of money the government proposes to spend during the respective fiscal year. In contrast, an appropriation bill is legislation that prescribes the amount of funding received by each respective program named in the federal budget.

During the budget process, each committee involved in composing the various budget bills will hear public testimony. This is an excellent opportunity to influence the amount of funding allocated to a specific program. **Table 2-6** presents some budget terminology. **Figure 2-3** outlines the budgeting process.

Table 2-6   Federal Budget Terminology

Appropriations Bill	Prescribes the amount of money dedicated to a respective program in the federal budget
Discretionary Spending	Funding that is not set each year, each year the funding level is debated and decided during the appropriations process
Entitlement Spending	This is mandatory spending, funding of these programs are required by law and must be funded in full each year
Reconciliation Bill	Legislation that balances federal revenue and expenses

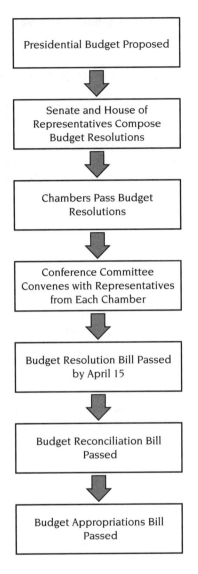

Figure 2-3   Federal budgeting process.

State Constitutions

Each state has its own state constitution. A state constitution is generally modeled after the US Constitution. The state constitution outlines the government structure of the state, and the powers and duties of each branch of government within the state. Generally, the governmental powers that are not designated to the federal government in the Constitution, nor prohibited by the Constitution, are reserved for the states or the citizens. **Table 2-7** presents the typical rules of law or policy content provided for in a state constitution.

Table 2-7   State Constitution Content

- Purpose of constitution
- Government purpose
- Outlines citizens' rights and due process
  - Property
  - Privacy
  - Intrusion
  - Expression
  - Religion
  - Assembly and petition
  - Voting
  - Fire arms
  - Discrimination
  - Jury, trial, prosecution, access to courts
- State sovereignty
- Distribution of power among branches of government
  - Defines legislative terms of office
  - Defines legislative process
  - Provides the structure and powers of the executive agencies
  - Appointment process of officials
  - Membership of boards and commissions
  - Judicial court structure and powers
  - Judicial procedures—appeals
  - Jury structure and selection
- Defines municipalities
  - Provides home rule charters and government plans
  - Local officials
  - Incorporation procedures
  - Inter-government cooperation
  - Election procedures

(continues)

Table 2-7   State Constitution Content (*continued*)

- Finance
  - ○ Power to tax
  - ○ Tax structure and base
  - ○ Tax approval process
  - ○ Revenue producing property
  - ○ Bonding
- Transportation
  - ○ Transportation system
  - ○ Funding
- Education
  - ○ Public education system
  - ○ Governance of education system
  - ○ Boards and commissions
- Natural resources
  - ○ As a revenue resource
  - ○ Protection of resources
- Policies regarding public officials and employees
- Code of ethics
- Police power
  - ○ Structure of state police
- Military power
- Methods to amend state constitution

City Charters

A city charter is a document that outlines a city's or municipality's governmental structure and laws. The city charter must be in alignment with the state constitution and US Constitution. A city charter is also known as a municipal charter. **Table 2-8** presents the typical outline of a city charter.

International Governing Bodies

The United States participates with other countries in governance structures that engage in international policymaking, for example, the World Health Organization and the United Nations.

Table 2-8   Components of a City Charter

- Preamble or purpose
- Defining of geographical boundaries and geopolitical units
- Office of mayor
- Government structure and powers
- City council
- District commissions or geographical organizational units and governance structure and power
- Budgeting process
- Local taxation
- City planning
- Defining of city property
- Public safety offices
  - Fire
  - Police
  - Medical/Emergency Systems
- Parks and recreation
- Executive agency departments—structure, power, and responsibilities
- Historical landmark developments and designation
- Local judicial system
- Local election
- Code of ethics

The World Health Organization (WHO) develops policy that directs and coordinates health initiatives within the United Nations system. WHO provides global leadership in health research agenda setting, establishing national guidelines and standards that are evidence-based, proposes multiple-policy options based on the best evidence, and provides technical support in assisting with the provision, monitoring, or assessment of health. The WHO has assumed shared responsibility for ensuring equitable access to health care and to defend against transnational threats to health and safety.

The United Nations is an international policy organization with a commitment to maintaining international peace and security, assisting development of friendly nations, promoting social progress, and supporting better standards of living. The United Nations engages in a multitude of activities that include but are not limited to peacekeeping, peace building, conflict prevention, humanitarian assistance, environmental and refugee protection, disaster relief, disarmament, protection of human rights, gender equality, economic development, promoting international health standards, and expanding food production. In addition, the United Nations supports the development of democratic systems. The United Nation's activities occur through a structure of five principal organs: General Assembly, Security Council, Economic and Social Council, Secretariat, and International Court of Justice.

Summary Points

- Government is an entity, organization, or institution that provides the structure of rule within a defined country or nation.
- The three primary functions of the United States Constitution are to allocate power between the federal government and the states (federalism), divide power among the three branches of government (separation of power), and limit the amount of government power (protection of individual liberties).
- The United States Constitution is the supreme law of the land
- Federalism separates the legal scope of authority into two governmental tiers, federal and state.
- The federalism structure sets up a hierarchy of powers.
- Total preemption exists when the federal government assumes all power over state laws.
- Partial preemption exists when a policy of the same or similar topic exists at the national and state levels.
- The three underlying principles of police power are to promote the greater public good, permit the restriction of private interest to promote public good, and permit pervasiveness of state powers.
- Parens patriae power provides the state with inherent power through sovereignty to safeguard citizens of the state.
- Governmental power and authority at the national level is shared among the three governmental branches—executive, judicial, and legislative
- Executive power is vested in the president of the United States.
- Judicial power is vested in the United States Supreme Court.
- Legislative power is vested in the United States Congress.
- The federal budget process is a collaborative effort between the executive and legislative branch of government.

- The federal budget fiscal year extends from October 1 through September 30.

References

Gostin, L. (2008). *Public health law: Power, duty, restraint* (2nd ed.). Los Angeles, CA: University of California Press.

Grad, F. (2004). *The public health law manual* (4th ed.). Washington, DC: American Public Health

Longest, B. (2005). *Health policymaking in the United States* (4th ed.). Washington, DC: Association of University Programs in Health Administration.

Mueller, D. (2001). Centralism, federalism, and the nature of individual preferences. *Constitutional Political Economy, 12*(2), 161–172.

Executive Branch: Federal Governmental Agencies and Appointed Bodies

The executive branch of the US government exercises policymaking powers through elected officials, official executive departments, and other executive-level agencies. The most powerful office in the executive branch is the office of the president of the United States. The US Constitution balances the power of the executive branch through the power bases of the legislative and judicial branches.

The Executive Branch Power Base

The executive branch of the government's powers is vested in the president of the United States. The president serves as the chief administrative or executive officer of the executive branch. As leader of the executive branch, the president serves as head of state, and commander in chief of the armed forces. In the United States, the president also serves as leader of all ceremonial functions. The primary responsibilities of the president are the development of policy; implementation and enforcement of policy by Congress; and appointment of his leadership team, the cabinet, and all heads of federal agencies.

The President

The American voters elect the president of the United States. In order to qualify for the presidential office a candidate must be at least 35 years of age, a natural born citizen of the United States, and resident in the United States for 14 years prior to the election. The president is elected through an electoral college system. The presidential election occurs on the first Tuesday in November of every fourth year. The population of the 50 states apportions the Electoral College. Each state provides an electoral member for each member of their congressional delegation, with the District of Columbia receiving 3 votes. The electors cast the votes for president on behalf of the American people. There are currently 538 electors in the Electoral College.

The president, as head of state, commander in chief, ceremonial leader, and head of governmental executive agencies leads the entire executive branch of government. The president appoints cabinet members who are responsible through delegated authority to manage and lead the operations of their respective executive agency. In addition to the cabinet, the Executive Office of the President (EOP) provides immediate staff support to the president.

The president is considered the chief policymaker in the United States and the most influential participant in the policymaking process. In addition to promoting national policy agendas, the president has the power to execute immediate policy in the form of an executive order. Other policy powers of the president are:

- Signing legislation into law or vetoing bills
- Negotiating and signing treaties (requires congressional ratification)
- Interpreting and clarifying existing laws for executive officers
- Extending pardons and clemencies

The president is constitutionally required to provide a State of the Union address to the American people. The president uses this opportunity to outline the executive branch's national policy agenda and to inform the American people of the impact of current national policies.

The Vice President

The election of the vice president occurs along with the president by the Electoral College. The vice president is considered the second in command. The vice president assumes the duties and responsibilities of the president if the president is unable to perform them. This might be permanent or temporary, and may be the result death, resignation, temporary incapacitation, or a vote of concern by the vice president and the majority of the president's cabinet regarding ability to function. The vice president serves as the president of the Senate. In the role of Senate president, the vice president can cast the deciding vote on the occasion of a tie vote. The daily oversight of the Senate is normally undertaken by the majority party leader.

Executive Office of the President

The Executive Office of the President (EOP) was developed in 1939 by President Franklin D. Roosevelt to facilitate the daily operations of the White House and presidential duties. The White House Chief of Staff is an advisor to the president and manages the entire EOP. The Office of the Press Secretary manages the White House Communications Office. The press secretary provides daily briefings to the media on behalf of the president to include policy issues and presidential activities. The National Security Council director advises the president on foreign policy, intelligence, and national security issues. Other councils or offices in the EOP include:

- Council of Economic Advisers
- Council on Environmental Quality
- National Security Council and Homeland Security Council
- Office of Administration
- Office of Management and Budget
- Office of National Drug Control Policy
- Office of Science and Technology Policy
- Office of the United States Trade Representative
- Office of the Vice President
- Executive Residence
- The White House

As an extension to the Executive Office of the President (EOP), there are several offices and departments within the White House that support the operations of the executive branch. These consist of:

- Office of Cabinet Affairs
- Office of the Chief of Staff
- Office of Communications
- Office of Energy and Climate Change Policy
- Office of the First Lady
- Office of the Social Secretary
- Office of Health Reform
- National Security Advisor
- Office of Legislative Affairs
- Office of Management and Administration
- Oval Office Operations
- Office of Political Affairs
- Office of Presidential Personnel
- Office of Public Engagement and Intergovernmental Affairs
- Office of the Press Secretary
- Office of Scheduling and Advance
- Office of the Staff Secretary
- Office of the White House Counsel
- Office of White House Policy
- White House Military Office

The President's Cabinet

The president's cabinet serves as an advisory body to the president and each cabinet member serves as the chief executive of their respective executive department. There are 15 cabinet members, generally members of the presidential succession line. The president's cabinet members are appointed by the president and confirmed by the Senate. The title of "secretary" is provided to each chief executive of a department, except the Justice Department, the head of which is the Attorney General. The 15 executive departments are:

- Department of Agriculture
- Department of Commerce
- Department of Defense

- Department of Education
- Department of Energy
- Department of Health and Human Services
- Department of Homeland Security
- Department of Housing and Urban Development
- Department of Interior
- Department of Justice
- Department of Labor
- Department of State
- Department of Transportation
- Department of Treasury
- Department of Veterans Affairs

The secretary of each department is directly responsible to the president. **Table 3-1** provides a summary of the duties of each department.

Table 3-1   Executive Department Policy Responsibilities

- Department of Agriculture (USDA)
  - Farming, agriculture, and food
  - Needs of farmers and ranchers
  - Promotes agricultural trade and production
  - Food safety
  - Protects natural resources and fosters rural communities
  - Focuses on hunger in America
- Department of Commerce
  - Promotes economic development
  - Promotes technological innovation
  - Supports business community
  - Issues patents and trademarks
  - Focuses on improving environment and oceanic life
  - Formulates telecommunications and technology policy
  - Promotes US exports
  - Enforces trade agreements
- Department of Defense
  - Deters war
  - Protects national security
  - Provides military forces

(continues)

Table 3-1   Executive Department Policy Responsibilities (*continued*)

- Department of Education
  - ○ Promotes academic achievement and preparation of students
  - ○ Fosters educational excellence
  - ○ Ensures equal access to educational opportunities
  - ○ Administers federal financial aid programs
- Department of Energy (DOE)
  - ○ Promotes energy security
  - ○ Supports development of reliable, clean and affordable energy
  - ○ Ensures nuclear security
  - ○ Protects the environment
- Department of Health and Human Services (DHHS)
  - ○ Protects the health of all Americans
  - ○ Provides essential human services
  - ○ Prevents disease outbreaks, assures food and drug safety
  - ○ Provides health insurance, administers Medicare and Medicaid
  - ○ Manages National Institutes of Health, Food and Drug Administration, and Centers for Disease Control and Prevention
- Department of Homeland Security
  - ○ Prevents and disrupts terrorist attacks
  - ○ Protects American people, infrastructure, and key resources
  - ○ Responds at the time of a national incident
  - ○ Patrols borders, protects travelers and transportation infrastructure
  - ○ Enforces immigration laws
  - ○ Promotes emergency preparedness
- Department of Housing and Urban Development (HUD)
  - ○ Develops national housing policy
  - ○ Improves and develops American communities
  - ○ Promotes home ownership and rent subsidy
  - ○ Enforces fair housing laws
  - ○ Provides mortgage and loan insurance
  - ○ Administers public housing and homeless assistance programs
- Department of Interior
  - ○ Protects natural resources
  - ○ Promotes recreational opportunities
  - ○ Protects fish and wildlife
  - ○ Honors responsibilities to native populations and cultures
  - ○ Manages dams and reservoirs
  - ○ Protects national parks and protected species
- Department of Justice
  - ○ Enforces laws
  - ○ Ensures public safety against foreign and domestic threats

(continues)

Table 3-1 Executive Department Policy Responsibilities (*continued*)

- ○ Provides leadership in preventing and controlling crime
- ○ Ensures fair and impartial justice for all Americans
- Department of Labor
  - ○ Ensures strong American workforce
  - ○ Job training programs
  - ○ Promotes safe working conditions
  - ○ Sets minimum hourly wage and overtime pay
  - ○ Ensures fair and equal employment opportunities
  - ○ Protects retirement and healthcare benefits
- Department of State
  - ○ Develops and implements president's foreign policy
  - ○ Counters international crime
  - ○ Provides assistance to US citizens and foreign nationals living or traveling abroad
  - ○ Promotes and maintains diplomatic relationships
- Department of Transportation
  - ○ Ensures safe and efficient transportation systems
- Department of Treasury
  - ○ Promotes economic prosperity
  - ○ Advises and enforces security of United States and international financial systems
  - ○ Produces nation's coins and currency
  - ○ Collaborates to promote global economic growth
  - ○ Predicts and prevents financial crisis
- Department of Veterans Affairs
  - ○ Administers veterans' benefit programs
  - ○ Operates veterans' medical care system
  - ○ Provides burial assistance
  - ○ Administers programs for veterans such as disability compensation, home loans, life insurance, rehabilitation

Executive Branch Independent Agencies

In addition to the departments in the executive branch that have representation in the president's cabinet, there are several independent agencies that are critical to the function of the executive branch of government. These administrative agencies are divisions of the government that enforce and administer policies in the form of laws and regulations. These independent agencies and their primary functions are outlined in **Table 3-2**.

Table 3-2   Independent Agencies Functions

- Central Intelligence Agency (CIA)
  - ○ Conducts counterintelligence
  - ○ Conducts foreign intelligence
  - ○ Maintains national security
- US Commission on Civil Rights
  - ○ Investigates complaints of discrimination
- Consumer Product Safety Commission
  - ○ Reduces risk of injuries and death from consumer products
  - ○ Formulates and enforces product safety standards
- Corporation for National and Community Service
  - ○ Supports the American culture of citizenship, service and responsibility
- Environmental Protection Agency (EPA)
  - ○ Protects human health and natural environment (air, water, and land)
- Equal Employment Opportunity Commission (EEOC)
  - ○ Promotes equal opportunity in employment
  - ○ Enforces federal civil rights laws
- Farm Credit Administration (FCA)
  - ○ Responsible for examining and regulating the Farm Credit System
- Federal Communications Commission (FCC)
  - ○ Regulates interstate and international communications by radio, television, wire, satellite, and cable
- Federal Deposit Insurance Corporation (FDIC)
  - ○ Insures bank deposits
- Federal Election Commission (FEC)
  - ○ Enforces Federal Election Campaign Act
- Federal Maritime Commission
  - ○ Responsible for the regulation of ocean-borne transportation in foreign commerce
- Federal Mediation and Conciliation Service (FMCS)
  - ○ Preserves and promotes labor management peace and cooperation.
- Federal Reserve System
  - ○ Ensures stable financial system
  - ○ Regulates credit conditions and loan rates
  - ○ Regulates banks
- Federal Trade Commission (FTC)
  - ○ Enforces federal antitrust and consumer protection laws
  - ○ Ensures capital system of healthy competition, free of unfair restrictions; and fair consumer policies
- General Services Administration (GSA)
  - ○ Provides government workplaces by constructing, managing, and preserving government buildings and by leasing and managing commercial real estate
  - ○ Offers private sector professional services, equipment, supplies, telecommunications, and information technology to government organizations and the military

(continues)

Table 3-2   Independent Agencies Functions (*continued*)

- International Trade Commission
  - Holds investigative responsibilities on matters of trade
  - Investigates the effects of dumped and subsidized imports on domestic industries and conducts global safeguard investigations
  - Adjudicates cases involving imports that allegedly infringe on intellectual property rights
- National Aeronautics and Space Administration (NASA)
  - Develops space exploration programs, artificial satellites, and rocketry
- National Archives and Records Administration (NARA)
  - Maintains National Archives
- National Endowment for the Arts (NEA)
  - Supports arts community
  - Funds museums, artists, and arts-related programs
- National Endowment for the Humanities
  - Supports research, education, preservation, and public programs in the humanities
- Director of National Intelligence
  - Integrates foreign, military and domestic intelligence in defense of the homeland and of US interests abroad
- National Labor Relations Board (NLRB)
  - Monitors relations between unions and employers in the private sector
  - Investigates unfair labor practices by unions and employers
- National Mediation Board
  - Facilitates labor-management relations within railroads and airlines systems
  - Endeavors to minimize work stoppages in the airline and railroad industry
- National Science Foundation (NSF)
  - Promotes science and engineering research, and educational programs
- National Transportation Safety Board (NTSB)
  - Investigates civil aviation, railroad, highway, and marine accidents
  - Develops transportation standards
- Nuclear Regulatory Commission
  - Licenses and regulates nonmilitary use of nuclear energy
- Office of Personal Management (OPM)
  - Recruits and retains government workforce
- Securities and Exchange Commission (SEC)
  - Administers federal securities laws
  - Protects investors in securities markets
- Selective Service System (SSS)
  - Provides human resources to the armed forces
- Small Business Administration (SBA)
  - Provides financial and technical assistance to promote business development
- Untied States Postal Service
  - Provides reliable, affordable, and universal mail service

Order of Presidential Succession

The Presidential Succession Act of 1792 outlines the order of succession to the presidency if the president should become incapacitated. This ensures continual functioning of the executive branch of government and protects the security of the American people and the country's infrastructure. The order of presidential succession is:

- Vice President
- Speaker of the House
- Senate President pro tempore
- Secretary of State
- Secretary of Treasury
- Secretary of Defense
- Attorney General (Department of Justice Secretary)
- Secretary of Interior
- Secretary of Agriculture
- Secretary of Commerce
- Secretary of Labor
- Secretary of Health and Human Services
- Secretary of Housing and Urban Development
- Secretary of Transportation
- Secretary of Energy
- Secretary of Education
- Secretary of Veterans Affairs
- Secretary of Homeland Security

Czar

The president of the United States has the authority to appoint officials who are responsible for specialized areas of policymaking. These individuals generally have a title associated with that specialized area. In the United States, the term "czar" has been used to refer to these individuals. The term czar is an informal title. At the time of appointment, the president determines the scope of authority and administrative responsibilities for the prospective czar. This appointment process is conducted as a measure to ensure efficient policymaking in areas of great concern or crisis.

Office of the First Lady of the United States

The spouse of the United States president administers the Office of the First Lady of the United States. The role and responsibilities of this office has evolved over time and changes with each First Lady. The First Lady has her own personal staff to implement the activities of the Office of the First Lady. The typical functions of the First Lady and her staff are to serve as hostess for the White House, manage all social and ceremonial events of the White House, and represent her office regarding official state business. The staff of the Office of the First Lady includes but is not limited to a social secretary, chief of staff, press secretary, chief floral designer, executive chef, and other White House staff. The First Lady usually selects an area of interest in which to become involved on behalf of the American people. She might serve as a spokesperson, use her position to implement policymaking, and may engage in political activities that impact the policy agenda within this area of interest.

White House Fellows and Interns

The White House Fellows program provides young Americans with an opportunity to engage in policymaking activities in the executive office. The White House Fellows enjoy a full-time paid position working with White House staff, cabinet secretaries, and other executive officers. During their tenure, they engage in roundtable discussions and study domestic and international policy. Their responsibilities might include chairing interagency meetings, design and implementation of federal policies, drafting speeches for their executive officer such as a cabinet secretary, and agency representation on Capitol Hill.

In contrast, the White House intern is an unpaid position. A White House intern acquires leadership skills and professional experience in preparation for a future in public service. The intern performs duties as assigned with a focus on increasing their knowledge regarding the functions and policymaking of the executive branch.

Executive Offices: State and Local Governmental Level

A governor and mayor hold the chief executive offices at the state and local government level, respectively. In addition, some cities are further divided into municipalities or counties that have a similar elected official of the executive branch of government, for example, a county president. The managerial operational activities of elected officials at the state, city, or local level is analogous to those of the federal executive office. As a representative of the executive branch of government, these officials are responsible for administering laws, enforcing state constitutions or city charters, and serving as chief executive officer. **Tables 3-3** and **3-4** outline some responsibilities and duties of these elected chief executive offices at the state and local level.

Table 3-3   Gubernatorial Responsibilities

- Signs bills into state statue; may use line item veto if permitted by state constitution and law
- Executes executive orders
- Administers legislative recommendations
- Monitors activities of executive departments of the state government
- Provides legislature with general and fiscal information regarding the current "state of the state"
- Creates and submits an operating budget for state legislature approval
- Collaborates with state Board of Pardons, serves as the last court of resort
- Appoints and removes executive officials, members of boards and commissions
  - Generally requires state Senate confirmation
- Serves as commander in chief of state's military
- Convenes special legislative sessions
- Declares special elections
- Serves as official spokesperson for state

Table 3-4   Mayoral Responsibilities

- Submits city budget to city council for approval
- Appoints executives of city offices
- Appoints advisory committees and commissions
- Serves as official spokesperson for city
- Signs city ordinances into law or executes veto power
- Enacts ordinances, resolutions, and other legislative orders from city council
- Executes executive orders
- Recruits city business
- Executes official city contracts
- Manages city utility services
- Promotes city living
  - Promotes arts, cultural affairs, parks and recreation, tourism industry
- Engages in community activities
- May preside over city council meetings. May deliver tie breaking vote on city council.
- May call city council into special meetings
- Manages health and safety services in city
  - Fire department
  - Police department
  - Health department

Summary Points

- The executive branch of government exercises policymaking powers through elected officials, official executive departments, and other executive level agencies.
- President of the United States is the most powerful position in the executive branch.
- The president serves as the chief administrative or executive officer of the executive branch.
- The president, as head of state, commander in chief, ceremonial leader, and head of governmental executive agencies leads the entire executive branch of government.
- The president appoints cabinet members.
- The president is considered the chief policymaker in the United States and the most influential participant in the policymaking process.

- The vice president is considered the second in command.
- The vice president presides over the Senate.
- The president's cabinet serves as an advisory body to the president and each cabinet member serves as the chief executive of their respective executive department.
- The order of presidential succession is established by the Presidential Succession Act.
- The president of the United States has the authority to appoint officials who are responsible for a specialized areas of policymaking, sometimes known as a "czars."
- The typical functions of the First Lady and her staff are to serve as hostess of the White House, manage all social and ceremonial events of the White House, and represent her office regarding official state business.
- White House Fellows and interns engage in activities of the executive branch of government and may participate in various aspects of policymaking.

Legislative Branch: Role in Policy

T he legislative branch of government consists of elected officials that represent the citizens of the United States. The legislative branch of government is known as the Congress of the United States, and is comprised of two chambers: the House of Representatives and the Senate.

Legislative Structure: Congress of the United States

The role of the legislative branch in policymaking is the passage of public laws for the entire country. In the Congress, the legislative work of developing laws for our country is primarily accomplished through standing committees in each chamber. There are special committees in each chamber and joint committees with bicameral membership. The two chambers are considered to have equal voice in the development of policy and legislation. In the policymaking process, bills that are passed by each chamber must be signed by the president or governor prior to becoming law. These bills are required to be signed within 10 days or they become law automatically.

House of Representatives

The House of Representatives (House) is responsible for originating all revenue bills. The House of Representatives also holds the power to impeach the president and other federal officers. Every bill that originates within the House must also be passed and approved by the Senate. Reciprocally, the House must pass and approve every bill that originates in the Senate.

Senate

The United States Senate was created to function as a legislative body in which each state has equal representation. The Senate is considered the most powerful chamber or house of Congress. The Senate has the power to conduct the impeachment trial of a president. The Senate is considered the senior legislative body of the Congress. In addition to bill passage, other functions of the Senate include:

- Ratification of treaties
- Ratification of presidential or gubernatorial appointments
- Conducting impeachment trials once the House of Representatives passes a bill of impeachment
- Consenting to legal declaration of war

The vice president of the United States serves as the president of the Senate. The president of the Senate does not have a vote unless there is a tie. Senate presidency is the primary constitutional role of the vice president.

Political Parties

A democracy supports the ability of individuals and groups to affiliate with a political party. A democracy requires an informed citizenry that has the ability to openly and freely engage in debate on issues, problems, politics, and policy solutions. The US Constitution supports the engagement of democratic processes that permit all voices to be heard without fear of retaliation. Political parties provide the formal structure from which democracy is practiced. Political parties are "basic institutions for the translation of mass preferences into public policy" (Heineman, 1996, p. 121).

Political parties integrate the values and belief systems of a group of persons into governmental policy by establishing a policy platform. Heineman (1996) proposes that political parties provide three critical functions to our democracy: (1) to provide for the orderly transfer of power within the party to continually foster a specific policy agenda; (2) to offer policy alternatives consistent with the party values and beliefs; and (3) to serve as a vehicle of innovation and ideas for specific causes. The most prominent political parties in the United States are the Democratic Party and the Republican Party.

Democratic Party

The Democratic Party pledges a commitment to keeping our nation safe and expanding opportunity for every American. The Democratic Party's commitment is reflected in their party platform or agenda that emphasizes strong economic growth; affordable health care for all Americans; retirement security; open, honest and accountable government; and securing our nation while protecting our civil rights and liberties. To understand the political environment and the policies formulated by each respective political party, it is critical to have a basic understanding of their party platform or agenda. The Democratic Party platform includes:

- Renewing the American Dream
  - Jumpstart the Economy and Provide Middle Class Americans Immediate Relief
  - Empowering Families for a New Era
    - Affordable, Quality Healthcare Coverage for All Americans
    - Retirement
    - Good Jobs with Good Pay
    - Work and Family
    - Poverty
    - Opportunity for Women
  - Investing in American Competitiveness
    - New American Energy
    - A World Class Education for Every Child
    - Science, Technology, and Innovation
    - Invest in Manufacturing and Our Manufacturing Communities
    - Creating New Jobs by Rebuilding American Infrastructure
    - A Connected America

- Support Small Business and Entrepreneurship
- Real Leadership for Rural America
  o Economic Stewardship
    - Restoring Fairness to Our Tax Code
    - Housing
    - Reforming Financial Regulation and Corporate Governance
    - Consumer Protection
    - Savings
    - Smart, Strong, and Fair Trade Policies
    - Fiscal Responsibility
- Renewing American Leadership
  o Ending the War in Iraq
  o Defeating Al Qaeda and Combating Terrorism
    - Win in Afghanistan
    - Seek a New Partnership with Pakistan
    - Combat Terrorism
    - Secure the Homeland
    - Pursue Intelligence Reform
  o Preventing the Spread and Use of Weapons of Mass Destruction
    - A World without Nuclear Weapons
    - Secure Nuclear Weapons and the Materials to Make Them
    - End the Production of Fissile Material
    - End Cold War Nuclear Postures
    - Prevent Iran from Acquiring Nuclear Weapons
    - De-Nuclearize North Korea
    - Biological and Chemical Weapons
    - Stronger Cyber-Security
  o Revitalizing and Supporting Our Military, Keeping Faith with Veterans
    - Expand the Armed Forces
    - Recruit and Retain
    - Rebuild the Military for 21st-Century Tasks
    - Develop Civilian Capacity to Promote Global Stability and Improve Emergency Response
    - Do Right by Our Veterans
    - Lift Burdens on Our Troops and Their Families
    - Restore the Readiness of the Guard and Reserve
    - Allow All Americans to Serve
    - Reform Contracting Practices and Make Contractors Accountable

- ○ Working for Our Common Security
  - • Support Africa's Democratic Development
  - • Recommit to an Alliance of the Americas
  - • Lead in Asia
  - • Strengthen Transatlantic Relations
  - • Stand with Allies and Pursue Diplomacy in the Middle East
  - • Deepen Ties With Emerging Powers
  - • Revitalize Global Institutions
- ○ Advancing Democracy, Development, and Respect for Human Rights
  - • Build Democratic Institutions
  - • Invest in Our Common Humanity
  - • Global Health
  - • Human Trafficking
- ○ Protecting our Security and Saving our Planet
  - • Establish Energy Security
  - • Lead to Combat Climate Change
- • Renewing the American Community
  - ○ Service
  - ○ Immigration
  - ○ Hurricane Katrina
  - ○ Preventing and Responding to Future Catastrophes
  - ○ Stewardship of Our Planet and Natural Resources
  - ○ Metropolitan and Urban Policy
  - ○ Firearms
  - ○ Faith
  - ○ The Arts
  - ○ Americans with Disabilities
  - ○ Children and Families
  - ○ Fatherhood
  - ○ Seniors
  - ○ Choice
  - ○ Criminal Justice
  - ○ A More Perfect Union
- • Renewing American Democracy
  - ○ Open, Accountable and Ethical Government
  - ○ Reclaiming Our Constitution and Our Liberties
  - ○ Voting Rights
  - ○ Partnerships with States

    o Invest in Social Innovation and Ideas That Work
    o Tribal Sovereignty
(Democratic National Convention Committee, 2008)

Republican Party

The Republican Party supports the individual over the government. This party advocates reducing the size of government, streamlining bureaucracy, and returning power to the individual states. The primary Republican Party platform or agenda consists of:

- Defending our nation, supporting our heroes, and securing peace
  - o Homeland security
  - o Better intelligence
  - o Terrorism and nuclear proliferation
  - o Immigration, national security, and the rule of law
  - o Providing for the armed forces
  - o Fulfilling our commitment to our veterans
  - o Promoting human rights and American values
  - o Procurement reform
  - o Sovereign American leadership in international organizations
  - o Helping others abroad
  - o Strengthening ties in America
  - o Advancing hope and prosperity in Africa
  - o Partnerships across the Asia-Pacific region
  - o Strengthening our relationship with Europe and Middle East
- Reforming government to serve the people
  - o Control spending
  - o Improve oversight of government programs
  - o Empowering the states, improving public services
  - o Improve the work of the government
  - o Domestic disaster response
  - o Restoring our infrastructure
  - o Entitlement reform
  - o Appointing constitutionalist judges for the nation's court
  - o Protecting the right to vote in fair elections
  - o Conduct a census
  - o Working with American territories
  - o Preserving the District of Columbia

- Expanding opportunity to promote prosperity
  - Republican tax policy—use tax relief to grow the economy
  - Small businesses as growth engines
  - Develop a flexible innovative workforce
  - Technology and innovation
  - Protecting union workers
  - Rebuilding home ownership
  - Reform the civil justice system
  - Free and fair trade
  - Support agricultural communities
- Energy independence and security
  - Grow energy supply
  - Reduce fossil fuel demands
- Environmental protection
  - Addressing climate change responsibility
  - Maintain stewardship over environment
- Healthcare reform: Putting patients first
  - Do no harm as the first principle
  - Patient control and portability
  - Improve quality of care and lower cost – end a sick care system
  - Fund medical research
  - Protecting rights of conscience
  - Building a healthcare system for future emergencies
- Education means a more competitive America
  - Early childhood education
  - Access to best teachers
  - Assert family rights in schools
  - Meeting college cost
  - Review federal role in education
  - Critical role of community colleges
- Protecting our families
  - Stop online child predators and end child pornography
  - Internet gambling
  - Rid the nation of criminal street gangs
  - Lock up criminals
  - Protect law enforcement officers
  - Reforming prisons and serve families
  - Improve law enforcement

o Continue the fight against illegal drugs
o Secure our civil liberties
o Protect victims of crimes
o Renew neighborhoods and build communities
o Preserving our values
o Constitutional right to bear arms
o Ensure equal treatment for all
o Protecting our Nation's symbols
o Freedom of speech and press
o Maintaining the sanctity and dignity of human life
o Preserving the traditional marriage
o Safeguard religious liberties
o Preserve American's property rights
o Support Native American communities
(Republican National Convention Committee, 2008)

Role of Congressional Members

Members of Congress engage in the entire policymaking process. Congressional members must be well informed regarding multiple issues and be ability to generate multiple policy alternatives as well as take firm policy positions. **Table 4-1** presents the role and responsibilities of congressional members. The manner in which a congressional member approaches policymaking is dependent upon their decision-making ability. Congressional members who support the basic tenet of *bounded rationality* perceive that policymaking processes and the respective political actions are intentionally rational in nature and follow a linear procedural process. S*ubstantive rationality* assumes complete rationality in which the congressional member has complete information prior to making a decision, weighing the pros and cons of each policy alternative solution. P*rocedural rationality* uses mental shortcuts to process incoming policy information and engage in decision-making processes (Smith & Larimer, 2009).

Regardless of which cognitive processes are employed to generate policies, most policymakers are not fully rational. This lack of rationality results from congressional members having to engage in policymaking activities without complete information, and having limited policy and political perspective

Table 4-1   Congressional Officers Roles and Responsibilities

Senate Officers

Role	Responsibilities
President	Role of vice president Casts a tie-breaking vote Makes parliamentary decisions which may be overturned by a majority vote
President Pro Tempore	Presides in absence of president of Senate Most senior or highest ranking senator
Presiding Officer	Member of the majority party Maintains order and decorum Recognizes members to speak Interprets the Senate's rules, precedents, and practices
Sergeant at Arms	Chief security officer Preserves order
Secretary	Chief legislative officer Elected by full Senate Affirms accuracy of bill text Supervises all printing of the bills, reports, and publications
Secretary for the Majority	Nominated by the majority leader and approved by the majority party Supervises phone directory, messengers, organizes meetings Briefs senators on votes and pending legislation Conducts all polls
Secretary for the Minority	Nominated by minority leader Responsibilities are analogous to secretary of the majority

United States House of Representatives

Role	Responsibilities
Clerk of the House	Presides at opening of Congress Receives credentials of members Notes voting tally and certifying bill passage Formal preparation of all legislation Maintains and distributes documents

(continues)

Table 4-1   Congressional Officers Roles and Responsibilities (*continued*)

United States House of Representatives

Role	Responsibilities
Director of Non-Legislative & Financial Services	Operational and financial responsibility Oversees House post office and finance office
Doorkeeper of the House	Arranges for joint sessions and joint meetings of Congress Announces messages from president and Senate Announces the arrival of the president to address Congress
Speaker of the House	Presiding officer, elected by the majority party Appoints committee chairs, all special committees, and conference committees Primarily casts tie-breaking vote

Common Senate and House Officers

Role	Responsibilities
Committee Chairperson	Most senior member of the majority party assigned to that committee
Floor Leaders	Consist of the majority leader and the minority leader
Majority Leader	Elected by the majority party in each house to serve as the spokesperson Manage and schedule the legislative and executive business in the respective chamber
Minority Leader	Elected by the minority party in each chamber
Parliamentarian	Advises the Senate and House on the interpretation of parliamentary procedure
Ranking Member	Member of the party who has the most seniority
Whip	Legislator chosen to assist the leaders of the majority and minority parties to secure votes

to completely weigh all pros and cons of each policy alternative solution prior to decision making. Congressional members are assisted in the policymaking process by legislative staff. **Table 4-2** presents the typical responsibilities of legislative staff positions. In addition, **Figure 4-1** outlines a typical organizational chart for a congressional office.

Table 4-2   Staff Positions

Administrative Assistant (AA) or Chief of Staff (CoS)
- Manages the office operations
- Responsible for hiring
- Chief assistant to the congressional or legislative member

Legislative Assistant (LA)
- Analyzes legislation and the implications of the legislative policy change
- Provides policy briefings
- Works with other congressional or legislative assistants with the respective member's office and from other members' offices

Legislative Director (LD) or Senior Legislative Assistant or Legislative Coordinator
- Manages and coordinates the work of all legislative assistants

Press Secretary or Communications Director
- Handles media relations
- May write member's speeches
- Maintains contact with constituents through newsletters or other mediums of correspondence
- May maintain media coverage in home state, district, or local area

Appointment Secretary or Scheduler
- Schedules member's activities
- Exerts some control over member's calendar and access to member

Personal Assistant, Secretary, or Executive Secretary
- Provides clerical duties for member
- May assist with personal tasks

Caseworker or Constituent Services Representative
- Handles individual constituent needs and concerns
- Maintains communication between individual constituents and the member and member's other staff regarding constituent's needs and concerns

Legislative Correspondent
- Answers correspondence

Office Manager
- Handles the operational functions of the office without the political involvement of the administrative assistant
- Handles staff and scheduling of office workers, volunteers

Systems Administrator, Technology Administrator
- Maintains the office technology, networks, etc.

District Director, District Coordinator, or District Legislative Coordinator
- For congressional members, this individual manages legislative activities and office at home

Receptionist or Staff Assistant
- Greets visitors
- Answers phone
- May assist with managing member's email

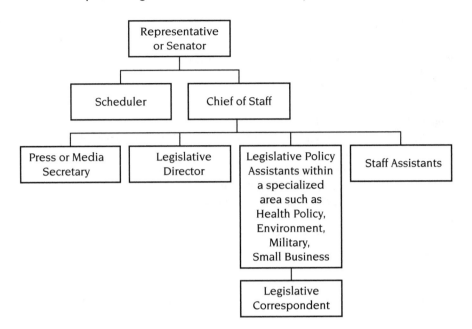

Figure 4-1   Sample organizational chart of congressional office staff

Formation of Law

The formation of law is rooted in the legislative process. Laws are generated through a process that is initiated with the composing of a bill. A bill can be composed by anyone but can only be introduced in a legislative body as a bill by an elected official such as a state legislator or congressional official. Legislators introduce bills for multiple purposes. For example, the intent when introducing legislation may not be the adoption of the bill in the form of a law, at a specific time. Legislators file bills as a medium in which to declare a position on an issue, to appease constituents or special interest groups, for publicity, or to demonstrate productivity as a member of Congress.

Once a bill is composed, it is sent to the clerk of the respective legislative chamber. The bill as this point is placed in a hopper. Often, legislation is introduced simultaneously in both chambers. However, a senator can postpone the introduction of a bill by a colleague by one day by voicing an objection. Every bill introduced in Congress has a lifetime of 2 years. The bill must be passed into law within 2 years or it dies by default. **Figure 4-2** outlines the formation process by which a bill becomes a law.

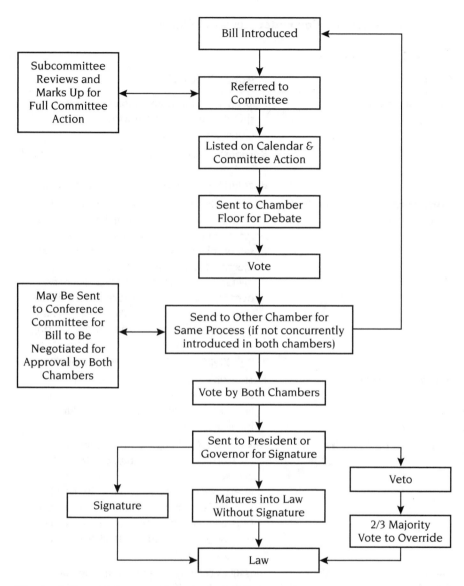

Figure 4-2   Legislative process: how a bill becomes law

Legislative Committees

Legislative committees form the framework of the policymaking process. **Table 4-3** presents legislative committee responsibilities. As each chamber of the legislature has rules and procedures for handling proposed bills, so does each legislative committee. Bills are referred to the respective committee for

Table 4-3   Legislative Committee Responsibilities

Senate Committees

Committee	Responsibilities
Appropriations	Appropriates funds and implements new spending under the authority of the Congressional Budget Act
Budget	Responsible for the federal budget, concurrent budget Resolutions and Congressional Budget Office
Commerce, Science and Transportation	Responsible for interstate commerce and transportation; Coast Guard; coastal zone management; communications; highway safety; inland waterways; marine fisheries; merchant marine and navigation; non-military aeronautical and space sciences; oceans, weather and atmospheric activities; inter-oceanic canals; regulation of consumer products and services; science, engineering and technology research, development and policy; sports; standards and measurement
Finance Committee	Responsible for health programs under the Social Security Act and health programs financed by a specific tax or trust fund; Medicaid; Medicare
Governmental Affairs	Responsible for budget and accounting measures; census and statistics; federal civil service; congressional organization; intergovernmental relations; District of Columbia; organization and reorganization of executive branch; postal service; efficiency, economy, and effectiveness of government; the United States archives
Health, Education, Labor And Pension	Measures relating to education, labor, health and public welfare; aging; biomedical research and development; Occupational Safety and Health, including the welfare of minors; private pensions plans; public health
Judiciary	Responsible for civil liberties; constitutional amendments; parental rights; family privacy
Special Committee on Aging	Issues that affect older Americans, including Medicare, prescription drugs, long-term care, and social security

(continues)

Table 4-3   Legislative Committee Responsibilities (*continued*)

House Committees

Committee	Responsibilities
Appropriations	Responsible for appropriation of the revenue for the support of the government; transfers of unexpected balances; new spending authority under the Congressional Budget Act
House Energy and Commerce	Responsible for biomedical research and development; consumer affairs and consumer protection; food and drugs; health and health facilities; interstate energy committee
Committee on Government Reform	Responsible for budget and accounting measures, generally; the overall economy, efficiency and management of government operations and activities, including federal procurement; public information and records; relationship of the federal government to the states and municipalities
Judiciary	Responsible for civil liberties; constitutional amendments; subversive activities affecting the internal security of the US
Transportation and Infrastructure	Responsible for federal management in emergencies and natural disasters; flood control and improvement of rivers and harbors; oil and other pollution of navigable waters, including inland, coastal and ocean waters; marine affairs (including coastal zone management) as they relate to oil and other pollution of navigable waters; roads and the safety thereof; transportation and transportation safety
Ways and Means Committee	Responsible for customs, collection districts, and ports of entry and delivery; reciprocal trade agreements; revenue measures; revenue measures relating to the insular possessions; bonded debt of the US; the deposit of public moneys; transportation of dutiable goods; tax exempt foundations and charitable trusts; national social security

action. *Standing committees* have permanent jurisdiction over specific types of bills. Some standing legislative committees have the authority to both authorize and allocate proposed laws. This concentrates a significant amount of power and influence over an issue within a specific committee. In contrast to a standing committee, the legislative leadership can appoint a *select committee* to manage a proposed problem or bill. A *joint legislative committee* is a committee that has representation from both the Senate and the House of Representatives. A *conference committee* is a type of joint committee that is typically assigned to work out differences in two respectively similar bills.

The leadership structure of a legislative committee consists of a committee chairperson and committee members. The chair of the committee is a member of the majority party. The chairperson is responsible for setting the agenda, conducting meetings, and managing the fiscal resources of the respective committee.

Legislative committees engage in a variety of critical activities. These activities are vital to the formation of policy. In addition, each of these activities serves as a point in the policymaking process at which constituents can influence the outcome of the proposed legislation. Typical activities in which committees engage include:

- Hearings—provide an opportunity for testimony; can be public or closed
- Legislation markup—markup is the process of editing, changing, or rewriting aspects of the proposed legislation or bill in public meetings, (in accordance with the "sunshine rules"), with national security or related issues being the only exceptions.
- Reports—outline the legislative intent of the bill, history of the bill, purpose and scope, changes proposed, fiscal impact, and sometimes summarize the dissenting opinions in relation to the proposed legislation

The legislative committee bears considerable responsibility for ensuring that proposed legislation reaches final passage into law. Potential committee actions are:

- Approve with or without amendments
- Rewrite or revise the bill
- Report the bill out to the full chamber favorably or unfavorably
- Take no action on the bill and let it die

Legislative Floor Action

Once the committee presents a bill, it can be placed on the calendar. The legislative body can take votes on a proposed bill by voice, division, or recorded voting. In *voice voting*, members stating their answer in support or opposition as either yea or nay. A *division vote* requires a head or hand count on the proposed legislation. A *recorded vote* records each legislator's name and position on the respective proposed legislation.

Executive Action

The executive leader (president, governor, or mayor) has the authority to sign, veto, or return legislation to the legislature with a detailed objection. If the executive leader does not take action within 10 days, the bill becomes law. If the legislature adjourns before the 10 day period expires, the unsigned bill does not become law by default. It is considered to be defeated by a *pocket veto*. If the executive leader vetoes a bill, it requires a two-thirds vote of Congress to overturn the veto.

Senate Confirmation

The United States Constitution requires that the Senate confirm the appointment of high government officials who are nominated by the president. The Senate confirmation process consists of three steps:

- Presidential nomination—The president submits in writing the name of a nominee. The nomination is read on the Senate floor and provided a number.
- Confirmation hearings—The Senate parliamentarian refers the nomination to the respective committee for review and confirmation hearings.
- Senate vote—The Senate reviews the committee's recommendation on the floor in a closed executive session. Nominations are open to unlimited debate. The Senate may confirm, reject, or take no action. Confirmation requires a simple majority vote. Once the Senate has acted, the secretary of the Senate communicates the decision, in writing, to the president. If the Senate is in recess for greater than 30 days or is in adjournment, the nomination must be returned to the president. During this time, the president can exercise a temporary appointment that ends at the conclusion of the Senate's next session unless the Senate confirms the appointment during the session.

Types of Law (Legal Policy)

There are four main types of law in the United States: constitutional; legislative; judicial or common; and administrative. Laws are established at the local, state, and federal levels. Law developed at the lower levels should not conflict with high level law and should be consistent with higher law. This is in accordance with hierarchical supremacy of a system of federalism. It is acceptable for laws developed at the lower level to be more specific than higher level laws providing they are consistent with national law. Law is considered a type of policy, typically referred to as legal policy. There are several types of legal policy that originate from our federalist structure. These are constitutional law, legislative law, and judicial or case law.

Constitutional law is the supreme law of the land. Constitutional law is derived from federal and state constitutions. The US Constitution establishes the general government of the nation and grants powers to the federal and state governments. The Constitution is the highest law that exists, and no other law can overrule it. The state constitution is the highest law at the state level, but can be invalidated by the federal constitution (Gostin, 2008).

Legislative law is developed through the legislative processes at the national or state level. Passage of laws by Congress or a state legislature results in legislative law or policy. These laws or polices are frequently known as *state statutes*. Local governing bodies such as city councils promulgate laws known as ordinances (Aiken, 2004).

Judicial law, or *common law* is also known as *case law*. Judicial law or policy is developed through decisions rendered in the judicial court system. Judicial law is founded on the principles of justice, reason, and common sense. Every decision made in a courtroom by a judge contributes to the development of judicial law. Judicial law can be either civil or criminal. Civil law protects individuals and enforces the rights, duties, and other legal relations that exist between private citizens. Criminal law consists of concerns that threaten society such as criminal or unlawful behavior toward another individual (Aiken, 2004).

As described in Chapter 3, executive agencies of the government promulgate regulations. Regulations are considered *administrative laws* or policies. Laws that are generated from regulatory agencies are known as regulations. In addition to developing regulations, executive agencies have police power to enforce these regulations.

Summary Points

- The legislative branch of government is known as the Congress of the United States.
- The Congress is composed of two chambers—the House of Representatives and the Senate.
- The House of Representatives is responsible for originating all revenue bills.
- House of Representatives also holds the power to impeach the president and other federal officers.
- Every bill that originates within the House must also be passed and approved by the Senate and vice versa.
- The Senate is considered the most powerful chamber or house of Congress.
- The vice president of the United States serves as the president of the Senate.
- A democracy requires an informed citizenry that has the ability to openly and freely engage in a debate on issues, problems, politics, and policy solutions.
- The most prominent political parties in the United States are the Democratic Party and the Republican Party.
- The Democratic Party pledges a commitment to keeping our nation safe and expanding opportunity for every American.
- The Republican Party supports the individual over the government, reducing the size of government, streamlining bureaucracy, and returning power to the individual states.
- Legislative committees form the framework of the policymaking process.
- Bills are referred to their respective committee for action.
- Standing committees have permanent jurisdiction over specific types of bills.
- A joint legislative committee is a committee that has representation from both the Senate and the House.
- A conference committee is a type of joint committee that is typically assigned to work out differences in two respectively similar bills.

- If the executive leader does not take action within 10 days, a bill becomes law.
- If the legislature adjourns before the 10 day period expires, the unsigned bill does not become law by default.
- The US Constitution requires that the Senate confirm the appointment of high government officials who are nominated by the president.
- There are four main types of law in the United States: constitutional, legislative, judicial or common, and administrative.
- Constitutional law is the supreme law of the land.
- Legislative law is developed through the legislative processes at the national or state level.
- Judicial or common law, also known as case law, is developed through decisions rendered in the judicial court system.

References

Aiken, T. (2004). *Legal, ethical, and political issues in nursing* (2nd ed.). Philadelphia, PA: F. A. Davis.

Democratic National Convention Committee. (2008). T*he 2008 democratic party platform*: *Renewing America's promise*. Retrieved from http://www.democrats.org/about/party_platform

Gostin, L. (2008). *Public health law: Power, duty, restraint* (2nd ed.). Los Angeles, CA: University of California Press.

Heineman, R. (1996). *Political science: An introduction*. New York, NY: McGraw Hill

Republican National Convention Committee. (2008). 2008 *republican platform*. Retrieved from http://www.gop.com/2008Platform/2008platform.pdf

Smith, K., & Larimer, C. (2009). T*he public policy theory primer*. Boulder, CO: Westview Press.

Judicial Branch: The Court System

The judicial branch is primarily responsible for the interpretation of legislation and policy, and the development of case law. Case law is considered legal policy. The courts, through the litigation process, are a means to enforce legislative and regulatory requirements. In addition, the litigation process uses the courts to enforce rights and responsibilities in accordance with legal policy.

Structure of Judicial Branch

The judicial branch is structured into two divisions in accordance with our federalist perspective. The two judicial branch divisions are federal courts and state courts. Each division also has lower courts (see **Figure 5-1**). The federal courts have jurisdiction over the US Constitution, and federal laws and regulations. Similarly, state courts have jurisdiction over the state constitution, and state laws and regulations. The supreme courts at the federal and state level are interconnected regarding appeals. An appeal of a state supreme court decision may be filed with the US Supreme Court. A Supreme Court decision is considered the highest legal decision that results in national policy for all citizens in our country.

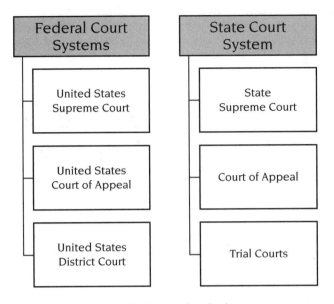

Note: Cases are generally initiated in the lowest court system and appeal upward to the highest court, such as the US Supreme Court or state supreme court.

Figure 5-1   United States court system

Federal Court System

The authority to create and abolish federal courts is established through the US Constitution. The only court that cannot be abolished is the Supreme Court. Generally, federal courts have jurisdiction over civil and criminal actions dealing with federal laws. The federal court is presided over by a federal judge appointee. The federal judge generally retains this appointment until death, retirement, or resignation. Federal judges are expected execute their duties with ethical behavior in upholding the law. Failure to do so may result in impeachment for improper or criminal conduct. The federal court system is administered by a chief judge or justice. The Clerk of Court maintains the courts records and finances. In addition, the Clerk of Court also provides support services, sends communications in the form of official notices and summons, and manages court reports and interpreters.

State Court System

The state court system interprets and enforces state laws under the auspices of the state government structure. State governments share power with a federal government. In accordance with the 10th Amendment to the US Constitution, all governmental powers not granted to the federal court system by the Constitution are reserved for the states and counties. **Figure 5-2** presents a typical state court system structure and function.

Special Court Systems

The US Congress has the authority to establish special legislative courts whose judges are appointed by the president and approved by the Senate for a life-long term. These special legislative courts are established through the legislative process. The two special courts that currently exist are the US Court of International Trade and the US Court of Federal Claims. In addition,

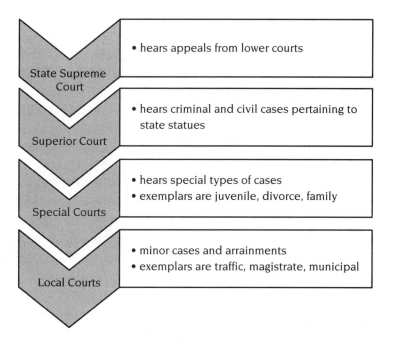

Figure 5-2   State court system structure and function

the US Attorneys or state attorneys general can exercise an unique system with which to bring forth a trial, known as a grand jury. In a grand jury, a jury convenes with government attorneys, court reporters, interpreters as needed, and witnesses to determine if there is sufficient evidence to indict an individual or "probable cause" that a suspect has committed a criminal act.

The US Court of International Trade has authority over cases involving international trade and customs. The US Court of Federal Claims has authority over claims for monetary damages alleged against the US government, disputes over federal contracts, or the unlawful seizure of private property by the government. A grand jury may be convened for cases involving charges of a federal or state level crime.

Jurisdiction

Jurisdiction represents the scope of authority for a case. There are several types of jurisdiction: geographic, subject matter, or personal. *Geographic jurisdiction* typically represents the geographic or political locality boundaries that are encompassed within the respective court's scope of authority. *Subject matter jurisdiction* concerns the specific area of law in which the respective court has a defined scope of authority. Lastly, *personal jurisdiction* is the extent to which a court has authority over an individual or business entity. For the purpose of disposing enforcement of legal policy on corporations, a corporation is treated as an individual in the federal and state judicial systems.

Litigation Process

The litigation process consist of three stages—the pre-litigation stage; litigation stage, which extends from the period of discovery to the point at which the case is heard before the court; and the post-litigation stage that attends to rendering the court's judgment and formulating the findings into future policy as case law.

Pre-Litigation Stage

The pre-litigation stage begins when an individual, usually a plaintiff, first meets with an attorney. The initial meeting with an attorney consists of an intake process that includes the following: (1) collection of personal data; (2) discussion of the complaints and allegations; (3) completion of necessary release forms allowing the attorney to represent the plaintiff; and (4) collection of supportive evidence in relation to the allegations.

Litigation Stage

The litigation stage is initiated when the first legal document is filed in the proper court jurisdiction. During this initial process, the case is assigned a docket number. The initial filing of documents for a legal case occurs in the court clerk's office. Typical initial documents that are filed might include: a summons, a complaint, an answer, interrogatives, requests for documents, subpoenas, and various motions. **Table 5-1** presents legal policy terminology used in the litigation process. An important aspect of the litigation stage is the discovery process.

Table 5-1   Terminology Used in Litigation Process

Affidavit	A written declarative statement provided under oath
Allegation	A legal assertion that must be proved or supported with evidence
Amicus brief	This is an unsolicited legal opinion provided by an *amicus curiae*, or "friend of the court," who is not party to a case. The court must grant permission for this information to be filed. This is a strategy often used by advocacy groups as a tool to advance certain opinions before the court.
Answer	A reply by the defendant or their attorney that states the manner in which the defendant intends to respond to the allegation
Arbitration	A binding process in which both sides agree to permit an external nonbiased arbitrator to render a decision on the disagreement or conflict
Breach	Failure to act in accordance with a duty
Class action	A case in which there are a large number of plaintiffs that pursue litigation under the same case and case number
Complaint	A legal document that sets forth the basic facts and reasons for the legal action

(continues)

Table 5-1   Terminology Used in Litigation Process (*continued*)

Cross examination	Questioning of a witness by the opposing side
Defendant	Person, company or institution against whom a claim or charge is filed
Depose	To have a deposition rendered
Direct cause	Act or event directly resulting in the injury
Discovery	Part of the pre-trial phase of litigation. The process by which evidence from the plaintiff and defendant is identified through securing documents and testimony such as a deposition.
Interrogatives	A set of written questions that must be answered
Jurisdiction	The boundaries that determines the scope of judicial authority
Malpractice	Deviation from accepted professional standards, by omission or negligence, that causes harm.
Mediation	A nonbinding process in which a mediator attempts to assist two opposing sides to reach a decision or settlement that is amenable to both parties
Motion for summary judgment	A request that the court provide an immediate ruling on behalf of the requesting party
Motion *in limine*	Motion "at the threshold." A motion made before the start of the trial, that certain evidence may or may not be presented during the litigation process
Motion to dismiss	A request that the court decide the case or render a decision; that there is no solution that could be rendered by the court
Motions	Legal documents filed by attorneys to facilitate the litigation process that request the court leader to make a decision on the case
Negligence	Failing to do something that should have been done, or doing something that should not have been done
Plaintiff	A person, company, or institution who files a suit in the court
Product liability	A product that is the cause of the injury that leads to litigation
Proximate cause	Causation in which an event that occurred prior to or immediately prior to an injury is associated with the injury

(continues)

Table 5-1   Terminology Used in Litigation Process (*continued*)

Request for document production	A written request in which one side requests the other side to produce documents that pertain to the case
Statue of Limitations	The time period in which the potential for litigation remains an option
Subpoena	A legal document that commands someone appear, testify, or produce a document
Subpoena *duces tecum*	A legal order for a person to appear at a deposition or trial and produce "tangible evidence" in the case
Summons	A legal document sent to the defendant that informs this individual that a legal proceeding has been initiated
Tort	A wrongful act in which another is injured, property is damaged, or reputation is harmed. Torts can be intentional or unintentional.
Tortfeasor	Person who commits a tort
Venue	Location or site of the court trial

Sources: Adapted from Aiken, T. D. (2004). *Legal, ethical, and political issues in nursing* (2nd ed.). Philadelphia, PA: F.A. Davis; Rudolph, E. G. (2009). *How to be a professional legal nurse consultant.* Memphis, TN: Jurex Center for Legal Nurse Consulting.

The discovery process seeks to identify the facts of the case, collect evidence, and gather other information supporting the case. It is during the discovery process that the attorney may file subpoenas, request documents, compose interrogatives, require physical or mental examinations, introduce admissions of fact, secure testimony and opinions of experts, and conduct depositions. The conducting of a deposition with the plaintiff, defendant, and experts is a critical element of the discovery process. A deposition is a formally structured interview process in which legal counsel from both sides are present with an individual providing the testimony under oath. A court reporter records the deposition verbatim. The deposition serves as evidence and can be entered in the court system during the litigation process (see **Table 5-2** and **Table 5-3**). The deposition is a source of evidence; therefore, it is critical that any individual who is deposed carefully read and correct the transcripts of the deposition. The deposition provides further leads for the continued investigation and discovery of evidentiary facts (Aiken, 2004; Rudolph, 2009).

Table 5-2   Deposition Purpose

A deposition during the litigation stage will enable the legal team to:
- Discover information regarding the facts of the case
- Evaluate the case's strengths and weaknesses
- Evaluate the knowledge of the witnesses
- Identify and develop a legal strategy
- Determine the relevance of documents to the case
- Discover the facts and circumstances of the allegation–complaint
- Preserve the testimony of a witness for a future date
- Determine the potential extent of injury
- Determine the credibility of potential witness
- Explore the extent of expert witness expertise
- Create evidence for trial

Table 5-3   Deposition Guidelines

The following are guidelines for an individual being deposed:
- Present a copy of your curriculum vitae (CV).
- Review all documents and pertinent information.
- Review any personal documentation regarding the incident.
- Review the format of the deposition with legal counsel prior to the deposition.
- Provide an honest testimony.
- Speak slowly, with clear pronunciation.
- Maintain eye contact.
- Answer only the question, do not elaborate on any questions or provide additional information not requested. Provide concise answers.
- Ask for clarification at any point if you do not understand the question.
- Always pause before answering a question to provide legal counsel with an opportunity to object.
- If asked the same question twice, answer in the same manner or request the recorder to read your previous answer.
- Avoid answering in an absolute manner, such as "I always ..." or "I have never. ..."
- Follow the lead of your legal counsel in answering questions.
- Do not provide speculations, only answer factual questions.
- If you do not know the answer, state "I do not know."
- If you do not recall or remember the events, state "I do not remember."
- Do not argue with legal counsel.

Another integral component of the discovery process is the conducting of legal research. Legal research produces valuable evidence to be utilized during the court litigation process. The purpose of legal research is to identify relevant case law that can provide guidance for legal strategy, assess the merits of the case, and identify judicial precedent in similar cases. During the legal research process the attorney or a designee conducts a comprehensive assessment of professional or scientific literature and reviews relevant case law that serves as legal policy (Aiken, 2004; Rudolph, 2009).

The final aspect of the litigation stage is the court trial in the judicial system. The trial is the hearing of the case in the presence of a judge. In some instance, the judge may hold pre-trial hearings to shorten the trial period. During pre-trial, the judge may render rulings on issues such as the qualification of witnesses, credibility of experts, admissibility of evidence, and response to motions filed. The trial consists of several phases such as jury selection, opening statements; presentation of evidence by the plaintiff's and defendant's legal counsel; closing arguments; judge's instructions to the jury, jury deliberations and findings of case, and verdict. In some cases, the court case is tried only in the presence of a judge.

Post-Litigation Stage

The jury or judge renders a final decision in each court case. This decision is know as the verdict. The decision or verdict rendered in response to a specific case formulates legal policy in the form of case law.

Types of Policy Formulated

Policy is formulated through the judicial system by the establishment of legal precedents and case law. This process is referred to as judicial policymaking. In judicial policymaking, the judge and court, acting as a collective entity, engage in an active role of policy implementation through the interpretive process. Case law in a system of jurisprudence is based on existing legal policy and judicial precedents. Case law is policy that is formulated through the judgment or verdict rendered in the judicial court system. Case law is also referred to as common law or judge-made law. Case law can define both civil and criminal policy within the respective jurisdiction of the judicial system.

A precedent is a policy that is established through an earlier judicial decision. *Stare decisis* or "let the decision stand," is the principle that establishes the basis for judicial precedence. This encourages adherence to previous case findings with substantially comparable facts and situations. Therefore, the development of case law serves as a precedent or policy by which future cases will be interpreted within the judicial system.

Nurses' Role in Judicial System

The effect of litigation within the judicial system is the establishment, affirmation, or clarification of rights at the local, state, or national level. Nurses can use their knowledge within the judicial system to serve as a legal nurse consultant or expert witness.

Legal Nurse Consultant

A legal nurse consultant is a professional who integrates nursing knowledge with knowledge of the legal system and process. The legal nurse consultant is as a member of the legal team. Legal nurse consultants are valuable resources who assist attorneys and judges in formulating legal policy. The duties of a legal nurse consultant include reviewing and evaluating medical–nursing legal cases, educating attorneys and clients regarding medical–nursing issues, reviewing and interpreting medical records, serving as an expert witness, testifying in a deposition or court, assessing the extent of damages, and conducting legal research (Rudolph, 2009). In addition, the legal nurse consultant can present a chronological summary of a case with an analysis of the case's merits in the form of an executive summary for the attorney or judge (Betts, Keepnews, & Gentry, 2006). This task expedites the rendering of a legal opinion or strategy.

Other healthcare professionals can integrate their discipline specific knowledge with the legal system and processes to serve as legal consultants. The legal nurse consultant model can be used to form a legal specialization within other healthcare professional disciplines. Nurses or other healthcare professionals can engage in the legal system as consulting experts or testifying experts. Both of these roles assist the attorney in determining the merits of the case and providing consultation regarding the legal case. However, there are differences in the role requirements. The consulting expert can provide consultation regarding their respective discipline and other areas involving the case. The consulting expert's information is not discoverable in the legal case unless it is used by an expert witness. In contrast, the expert witness provides testimony only in their scope of practice and their information is considered discoverable in a legal case. The role of the expert witness is further explained below.

Expert Witness

Nurses and other healthcare professionals serve as expert witnesses to provide information relevant to the case. An expert witness is an individual who has an identified area of expertise based on education, skills, credentials–qualifications, and experience (Aiken, 2004). Nurses who serve as expert witnesses generally provide testimony regarding the expected nursing standard of care within a healthcare environment. To be accepted as an expert witness, the nurse's or other healthcare professional's credibility in terms of education, experience, and credentials must be demonstrated by the team's attorney. The judge, on behalf of the judicial system, may then qualify the nurse or other healthcare professional as an expert witness in the court system.

Summary Points

- The judicial system is structured into two divisions—federal and state courts.
- The federal courts have jurisdiction over the US Constitution and federal laws and regulations.
- State courts have jurisdiction over the state constitution and state laws and regulations.
- An appeal of a state supreme court decision may be filed with the US Supreme Court.
- A Supreme Court decision is considered the highest legal decision.
- The only court that cannot be abolished is the Supreme Court.
- Federal courts have jurisdiction over civil and criminal actions dealing with federal laws.
- The federal court is presided over by a federal judge appointee.

- A federal judge generally retains appointment until death, retirement, or resignation.
- All governmental powers not granted to the federal court system by the Constitution are reserved for the states and counties.
- In a grand jury, a jury convenes with government attorneys, court reporters, interpreters as needed, and witnesses to determine if there is sufficient evidence to indict an individual or "probable cause" that a suspect has committed a criminal act.
- Jurisdiction represents the scope of authority for a case
- Geographic jurisdiction represents the geographic or political locality boundaries that are encompassed within the respective court's scope of authority.
- Subject matter jurisdiction concerns the specific area of law in which the respective court has a defined scope of authority.
- Personal jurisdiction is the extent to which a court has authority over an individual or business entity.
- The litigation process occurs in three stages: pre-litigation, litigation, and post-litigation.
- The judicial system produces policy in the form of legal precedents and case law.
- A precedent is a policy established through an earlier judicial decision.
- Case law is policy formulated through the judgment or verdict rendered in the judicial court.
- A legal nurse consultant is a professional who integrates nursing knowledge with knowledge of the legal system and process.
- An expert witness is an individual who has an identified area of expertise based on their education, skills, credentials–qualifications, and experience.

References

Aiken, T. D. (2004). *Legal, ethical, and political issues in nursing.* (2nd ed.). Philadelphia, PA: F. A. Davis.

Betts, V. T., Keepnews, D., & Gentry, J. (2006). Nursing and the courts. In D. Mason, J. Leavitt, & M. Chaffee (Eds.), *Policy & politics in nursing and healthcare* (5th ed., pp. 825–834). St. Louis, MO: Saunders/Elsevier.

Rudolph, E. G. (2009). *How to be a professional legal nurse consultant.* Memphis, TN: Jurex Center for Legal Nurse Consulting.

Public Health Policy

Public health law is a form of policy. As a form of policy, public health law is considered a population-based, community-level intervention that protects and maintains the public's health and safety. Public health law integrates concepts from law, medicine, health care, and public health (Gostin, 2008).

Public Health Law Defined

Definitions of public health law abound. The word "law" is frequently used to refer to the legal system, legal processes, the legal profession, and legal knowledge and learning. Public health law is defined within the context of public health policy, since public health law is considered public policy. Longest (2005) defines public health law as laws related to health, which can be enacted at any level of government. Gostin (2008) defines public health law as the legal powers and duties of the state that assure conditions of health for the people and limits the use of state powers to constrain autonomy, privacy, liberty, proprietary, or other legal protected rights of individuals.

Gostin's definition lists five essential characteristics of public health law: (1) the government is responsible for public health activities, (2) a population-based focus is assumed, (3) public health addresses relationships between the state and the population, (4) population-based services are delivered grounded in science, and (5) public health officers have the power to coerce individuals and businesses into actions that protect the health of the population (Gostin, 2008).

Foundation and Scope of Public Health Law

The scope of public health law is based on the hierarchy of legal power derived from federal constitutions, state constitutions, city charters, administrative regulations and judicial decisions. The US Constitution is the supreme law of the nation and reflects national values in relation to public health. At this level, public health laws are generated as a direct extension of the Constitution either through executive, legislative or judicial actions. For example, federal regulation by the Occupational Safety and Health Administration promulgates rules and regulations to safeguard worker safety and health based on federal legislation implemented through an executive agency.

The next level in the hierarchy occurs at the state level with the development of statutes. Similarly, these state statutes designed to protect the health of the general population may be formulated and developed in either the executive, legislative, or judicial branch of government.

Judicial decisions can generate public health policy. Judicial decisions are precedent-setting policy that generally interprets the intent of other policies developed through the executive or legislative branch. The courts also have the power to hold a statute or executive act null and void if it violates any law generated at a higher level in the federalist system, such as the state charter or the US Constitution. This is known as judicial review (Aiken, 2004; Gostin, 2008). **Figure 6-1** presents eight steps in the hierarchy of legal authorization in the United States.

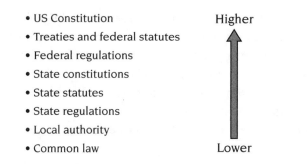

- US Constitution
- Treaties and federal statutes
- Federal regulations
- State constitutions
- State statutes
- State regulations
- Local authority
- Common law

Higher

Lower

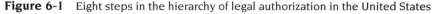

Figure 6-1   Eight steps in the hierarchy of legal authorization in the United States

Constitutional Law

Constitutional law originates from the US Constitution. Constitutional law outlines the limitations of power of, and the organizational structure for the United States government. Constitutional law provides individuals with fundamental rights and freedoms through its articles and amendments.

Public Health Laws

Public health laws focus on the health of the general population. Some public health laws are considered germane to the general health and welfare of the citizens of this country. The following public health legal policies are presented: individual rights, compulsory examination, quarantine and isolation, licensure and registration, inspection and searches, embargo and seizures, and nuisances.

Individual Rights: Due Process

An individual's rights are protected through the Bill of Rights in the US Constitution and bills of rights developed at state levels. The Bill of Rights in the Constitution consists of the first 10 amendments and a portion of the 14th Amendment. The 14th Amendment provides individuals with dual citizenship in the nation and their state of residence, entitling them to the rights outlined at the national and state level (Grad, 2004). The 5th and 14th Amendments prohibit the government from depriving individuals of life, liberty, or property, without due process of law (Gostin, 2008).

The due process clause provides two separate obligations: a substantive, and a procedural element. The substantive element requires the government to provide significant reasons and justifications for invading an individual's personal freedoms. The procedural element requires the government to provide an individual with notice and to ensure a fair process. The fair process consists of a notice, a hearing, and access to an impartial decision maker (Gostin, 2008). **Table 6-1** presents public health legal policy that protects the individual.

Table 6-1   Public Health Policy: Protection of Individual

Public health policy concept	Purpose, function, or policy intent (examples in parentheses)
1st Amendment	Freedom of religion, speech, press, and right of assembly (advertising cannot be misleading)
4th Amendment	Freedom from unreasonable search and seizure
5th Amendment	Protection against self-incrimination and double jeopardy (double prosecution or trial for the same offense, or two separate offenses that arise from one set of facts)
6th Amendment	Right to a speedy, public trial with an impartial jury, right to confront witnesses, right to counsel
8th Amendment	Freedom from cruel and unusual punishment
14th Amendment	Provides dual citizenship in the United States and state of residence
Right of privacy	Parts of our lives are not the government's business, freedom to seek or refuse treatment
Separation of religion and state	No law may interfere with religious beliefs (protection is limited if there is public concern); limits government's financial assistance to religious institutions or activities
Search and seizure	Permits search for evidence and seizure of evidence with an executed warrant; evidence gained with an illegal search or seizure is inadmissible in criminal proceedings
Violations of public health laws	Punishable as misdemeanors; can be tried separately under state and federal law if violation is both a state and federal crime (double jeopardy permitted)
Writ of *habeas corpus*	Judicial order; commands the jailer or other person detaining a prisoner to physically bring the prisoner before the court so that lawfulness of the detention can be determined

Compulsory Examination

Compulsory examinations are considered mandatory medical examinations. These require careful consideration and justification. The right to refuse treatment is embedded in ethical principles. Public health laws or policy may override the common law and authorize mandatory examination and treatment.

States support the public health provision for compulsory examination and treatment based on three interests: health preservation, harm prevention, and preservation of effective therapies (Gostin, 2008). Public health officers have statutory authority for compulsory examination if there is sufficient belief that a communicable disease exists; a compulsory examination cannot be based on mere suspicion (Grad, 2004). Compulsory examination can be mandated as a requirement for licensure, which is considered a privilege, such as testing for sexually transmitted disease prior to the issuance of a marriage license. In the presence of an epidemic, public health officials can require compulsory examinations, without concern for due process (Grad, 2004). **Table 6-2** presents public health legal policy that may restrict individual freedom to preserve the public's health.

Quarantine and Isolation

Quarantine policy originates principally from local and state powers. The states' power to quarantine is preempted by federal law pursuant to the federal government's power over commerce. The First International Quarantine Rules were adopted in 1852. The current promulgation of international quarantine laws originates from the World Health Organization (Gostin, 2008).

Quarantine orders must be based on reasonable belief, not merely suspicion. The enforcement of a quarantine policy consists of complete restriction of a person or persons to a specific location (Grad, 2004). This is generally enacted as a measure to prevent the transmission of communicable diseases. In contrast, isolation is the separation of individuals with a communicable infectious illness from the general public during the period of communicability (Gostin, 2008).

Table 6-2   Public Health Policy: Restrictions of Individual or Goods

Public health policy concept	Purpose, function, or policy intent
Compulsory examination	Required examinations such as in cases of communicable diseases or periodic screenings, or threatened epidemic; does not violate individual liberty or privacy if there is sufficient justification
Isolation and quarantine	Can quarantine individuals for some communicable diseases; complete restriction of the person and possibly household contacts; misdemeanor to break quarantine or to destroy the quarantine sign; can impose on the basis of reasonable belief; some states require actual order of confinement in the form of a warrant issued by a magistrate; public health official not liable if measures taken in good faith
Emergency commitment (mental illness)	To allow the state to provide emergency assistance to an individual; must be based on recent specific act, threat, or behavior of omission; examination must occur within a specified time period; supported by a written physician statement; generally valid for 48 to 72 hours
Committed individuals	Right to prompt and adequate humane treatment; right to reasonable safety, use of less restrictive measures; need a preponderance of evidence indicating there is no longer a danger present before release
Embargo	An order prohibiting the removal or use of items by affixing a tag or marking on the goods warning that it must not be removed; purpose is to prevent the dissemination of dangerous goods; owner has right to due process
Condemnation	Typically used with an embargo or seizure; an order for the destruction, denaturing, sale or re-exportation of goods or return to owner carried out by court proceedings; cost of destruction is the responsibility of the owner

Licensing and Registration

A licensure is a privilege extended to an individual or institution for a specific purpose. Licensure power originates at the local or state government level. Licensure process is initiated through the passage of legislation that prohibits certain acts without the possession of a license to engage in the specified activities (Grad, 2004). Licensure power permits an executive agency of the government to promulgate rules and regulations governing certain prohibited acts. The acceptance of a license by an individual or institution implies consent to submit to the conditions of the regulatory agency. A license is formal permission by an executive agency through the delegated authority to engage in specific acts not allowed to those without the license (Gostin, 2008). **Table 6-3** presents public health legal policy for institutions, businesses, or environments that preserves the public's health.

The licensure process establishes a system of continued monitoring and supervision for the purpose of protecting the public's health, safety, and welfare (Gostin, 2008; Grad, 2004). Licensure provides an individual with property rights and ensures the right to procedural due process. Licenses can be denied, suspended, or revoked; however, these disciplinary actions require a clear notice to the affected party, a hearing, a right to counsel, a right to secure evidence by subpoena, and the right to confrontational cross-examination of an accuser (Grad, 2004). Licensure cannot be suspended or revoked without proper due process.

Registration is a process of identification of and record keeping on certain individuals. Registration is simply a listing, while licensure specifies requirements that must be satisfied prior to being licensed (Grad, 2004). A registry is a listing without any pre-established conditions.

Search and Inspection

A *search* occurs when an official is looking for conditions that violate laws or, for instruments that may have been used in criminal activity. An *inspection* is a visitation or survey to determine if conditions that are deleterious to the public's health exist. Inspection does not include the aim of uncovering criminal evidence. Inspections are generally conducted on a routine basis and involve an evaluation for compliance with public laws or policies. The 14th Amendment provides protection from unreasonable searches (Grad, 2004).

Table 6-3 Public Health Policy: Institutions, Businesses or Environment

Public health policy concept	Purpose, function, or policy intent
Licensure	Permission to operate within the defined rules and regulations of the license; a condition of accepting the license is consent to continuing control of the regulatory agency; licensure does ensure due process rights
Searches and inspections (also known as administrative searches)	Search implies looking for particular conditions that constitute a violation of the law; Inspection is a visitation or survey to determine whether or not conditions deleterious to the health and welfare of the public exist; must be a supporting statue for the search or inspection
Exclusionary rule	Evidence seized during an administrative inspection usually cannot be used in criminal proceedings
"Plain view" doctrine	Evidence of criminal activity inadvertently discovered in the course of a legitimate public health inspection or other administrative search can be admissible if in plain view during the search or inspection activity
Public nuisance	An offense against the public; characterized by an interference with the public right to pursue normal conduct of life without threat to health, comfort, or repose; defined by statues or ordinances
Private nuisance	Interference with the use or enjoyment of private property; subject to damages by tort law; injunctions to stop interference
Violations order	An administrative order from a public health official or agency informing property owner of the existence of a lawful violation
Orders to abate	Order to stop the activity or condition creating a violation
Order to cease and desist	Order to end the prohibited condition
Compulsory disclosure	Must be permitted by law; power to require reports, inspect books, records or premises

Administrative search warrants are generally required to inspect residential and private commercial facilities (Gostin, 2008). However, a public health official can conduct a search if there is a legislative statute that provides the authority for such activity. An inspection or search without a warrant can be conducted under three conditions: (1) legally valid consent justifies an administrative search; (2) in an emergency to avert any immediate threats to the public's health or safety; and (3) under the "open fields" doctrine by which a public health office may search a public place. Pervasively regulated businesses, such as the food industry and health care, forfeit some rights of privacy and are subject to routine searches. Inspections are permitted without a warrant for a licensed business with a substantial public health significance. The acceptance of some licenses by businesses waives their right to privacy and permits public health officials to conduct routine searches. Public health officials can secure a search warrant by merely demonstrating specific evidence of an existing violation in health or safety regulations, or for a valid reason that is in the public health's interest (Gostin, 2008). Most states require a search warrant issued by a judge (Grad, 2004). Evidence secured during an administrative inspection cannot be used in criminal investigations unless the evidence was in plain view during the inspection. The "plain view" doctrine allows criminal evidence to be used if the evidence was in plain view of the public health inspector during the search (Grad, 2004).

Embargo and Seizure

Articles or items are *embargoed* by tagging or marking the article with a statement such as "this article is in violation of the law" (Grad, 2004). An embargo prohibits further use or removal of the identified articles. An embargo is placed when the articles are considered to pose a public health threat, as in the case of dangerous dissemination of contaminated or potentially infected goods. An embargo is a public health preventive measure. In contrast to embargo, *seizure* takes possession of goods that belong to another (Grad, 2004).

Nuisances

A *private nuisance* is the unreasonable interference with the use or enjoyment of private property (Gostin, 2008; Grad, 2004). Private nuisances are subject to tort law, and injunctions can be issued to stop the interference. A *public nuisance* is unreasonable interference with the community's use and enjoyment of a public place; or interference with the right to pursue the normal conduct of life, without a threat to health, comfort, or repose (Gostin, 2008; Grad, 2004). Public nuisance is typically defined by local ordinances or statutes. Public nuisances are subject to legal action by injunction or criminal prosecution.

The cessation of a public nuisance is fundamental to maintenance of a healthy environment. The following policy strategies can be implemented in order to stop the public nuisance:

- *Summary abatement order.* This order directs action to remove the offending condition prior to a hearing or court authorization. A summary abatement order is justified if there is significant and imminent risk or threat to the public's health.
- *Violations order.* This is an administrative order from a state or federal health officer or agency that informs the property owner of a legal violation.
- *Order to abate.* An order to abate requires the cessation of an activity or condition within a time period detailed in the order. The time period typically provides the individual with a "reasonable amount of time" to stop the activity.
- *Order to cease and desist.* This is an order to end a prohibited condition.
- *Injunction.* This is a court order that directs a person to perform a specific activity or refrain from engaging in a specific activity (Grad, 2004).

Personal Health Law and Policy

Personal health law is the scope of law that deals with individual persons and family health. Personal health law includes personal health insurance policies and laws governing personal injury. In addition, personal health law includes laws that provide legal guidance with regard to an individual's access to healthcare services. Laws that pertain to the impact that other individuals or the environmental may have on an individual's health are also considered a type of personal health law.

Environmental Health Law

Environmental health law is the scope of law that provides legal guidance concerning human impact on the environment and natural resources, and also the impact of the environment on humans. Environmental health law includes legal guidance regarding the use and disposal of toxic substances. In addition, environmental health laws provide guidance regarding our personal living space such as radon exposure levels, within our homes.

Occupational Health Law

Occupational health law is the scope of law that provides legal guidance regarding an individual's work environment. The Occupational Safety and Health Administration (OSHA) is the executive agency that primarily develops occupational regulations to protect the employee within the work environment. The Occupational Safety and Health Act provides the legal authority for OSHA to develop regulations governing the workplace.

Statutory Law

Statutory law is based on formal statues. Statues are written laws enacted by the federal, state or local legislative bodies. Federal statues are published and codified in the United States Code. Congress and state legislatures enact acts and statues. In contrast, at the local level, counties or parishes enact ordinances. These enactments govern human behavior, provide access to programs, and restrict certain activities that negatively impact individuals and groups. All statues or ordinances must be consistent with the respective state's constitution and the US Constitution.

Administrative Law

In the executive branch of government, executive-level agencies and organizations act within the scope of administrative law to enact their missions. Administrative laws exist at both the federal and state level to govern the practice of executive agencies. Administrative Procedure Acts exist at both the federal and state level that outline the legal procedures of administrative law. Administrative law provides basic procedural safeguards for federal and state regulatory systems and defines the scope of judicial authority over the federal or state agencies.

Administrative laws outline the process of developing regulations within the respective executive agencies. The rules and regulations developed by executive agencies are subject to challenge. These challenges are typically based on procedural rather than substantive grounds. The judicial system has deferential preference to the respective executive agencies' expertise and are unlike to interfere with the substantive decision rendered by the executive agency. However, procedural challenges are heard especially if there is concern with interference with an individuals basic constitutional rights. The judicial system can also be engaged in the legal process within the scope of administrative law if an executive agency has been requested to act and it did not act. The judicial system could be requested to render a judicial review and decision.

The executive agency acting within the scope of administrative law must maintain consistency with constitutional law and relevant statues and judicial precedence. Judicial review of an executive agency would take into consideration the following:

- Extent to which the executive agency stayed within constitutional and statutory authority
- Proper interpretation of applicable laws and statutory language
- Proceedings were conducted in a fair manner ensuring the individual's right to due process
- Rendered decisions are not arbitrary, capricious, or unreasonable
- Rendered decisions are based on substantial evidence

Tort Law

A tort is a wrongful act that creates harm. The idea behind tort law is that the harm or injury that occurs as a result of a wrongful act can be compensated, and that antisocial behavior is discouraged. Intentional torts are intentional or willful acts that violate another person's rights or property resulting in some type of harm. The primary factor of relevance in an intentional tort is the individual's intent in the action. Intent implies that the person acted for the purpose of causing or inflicting injury. The motive or purpose of the act has a critical role in determining the amount of liability resulting from the act. There are several types of intentional torts which include: assault and battery, false imprisonment, intentional infliction of emotional stress, and land trespass (Aiken, 2004).

Assault is the threat or attempt to inflict effective physical contact onto another person. Battery is the invasion of another person's privacy by unpermitted touch. False imprisonment is the unlawful and intentional confinement of another person within fixed boundaries in which the person is harmed by this confinement. Intentional infliction of emotional stress is the invasion of another person's peace of mind. Land trespassing is the unlawful interference with another person's possession of land by intruding on their property, failing to leave their property, or placing something on their property (Aiken, 2004).

In an intentional tort, the individual committing the tortuous act had requisite knowledge and the will to commit the wrongful act. In contrast, a non-intentional tort occurs when negligent conduct results in harm to another person. Negligence is failing to act when an individual should have acted to prevent harm to another person (Aiken, 2004). Negligence is based on the provision of prudent care. Therefore, negligence consists of doing something which another prudent healthcare professional would not do or failing to do something that another prudent healthcare professional would have done under the same or similar circumstances.

A third type of tort is quasi-intentional tort. A quasi-intentional tort results from the spoken word and includes: defamation, invasion of privacy, and breach of confidentiality. Defamation is the oral or written communication to a third party about a person that is false with the intent to injure that person's reputation. Slander is defamation using oral communication and libel is defamation using written communication. Invasion of privacy violates another person's right to be alone without the unreasonable interference of their personal life. Breach of confidentiality is providing an individual's private information to other parties without their expressed consent (Aiken, 2004).

Summary Points

- Public health law is a form of policy.
- Public health law is considered a population-based, community-level intervention that protects and maintains the public's health and safety.
- Law is frequently used to refer to the legal system, legal processes, the legal profession, and legal knowledge and learning. Public health law is defined within the context of public health policy, since public health law is considered public policy.

- Public health law can be defined as the legal powers and duties of the state that assure conditions of health for the people and limits the use of state powers to constrain autonomy, privacy, liberty, proprietary, or other legal protected rights of individuals.
- The US Constitution is the supreme law of the nation and reflects national values in relation to public health.
- Constitutional law outlines the limitations of power of, and the organizational structure for the United States government.
- The Bill of Rights in the Constitution consists of the first 10 amendments and a portion of the 14th Amendment.
- The 14th Amendment provides individuals with dual citizenship in the nation and their state of residence, entitling them to the rights outlined at the national and state level.
- The 5th and 14th Amendments prohibit the government from depriving individuals of life, liberty, or property, without due process of law.
- The due process clause provides two separate obligations: a substantive and a procedural element.
- Compulsory examinations mandate a medical examination.
- States support the public health provision for compulsory examination and treatment based on three interests: health preservation, harm prevention, and preservation of effective therapies.
- Quarantine and isolation are enacted to prevent the transmission of communicable diseases.
- A license is a privilege extended to an individual or institution to engage in specific activities that are legally protected.
- Registration is a process of identification of, and record keeping on, certain individuals. It is a listing or roster.
- A *search* occurs when an official is looking for conditions that violate laws, or for instruments that may have been used in criminal activity.
- An *inspection* is a visitation or survey to determine if conditions that are deleterious to the public's health exist.
- Search warrants are usually issued by a judge.
- Embargo and seizure prohibits the use or removal of materials as a measure to protect the public's health.
- Nuisances interfere with another's property or right to enjoyment.
- Environmental health law is designed to protect and preserve environmental resources.
- Occupational health law governs the workplace environment.

- Statutory law is based on formal statues which are written laws enacted by federal, state or local legislative bodies.
- Administrative law governs the activities of executive-level agencies.
- Tort law governs wrongful acts that create harm to another.
- Assault and battery are torts.
- Torts can be intentional or unintentional.

References

Aiken, T. D. (2004). *Legal, ethical, and political issues in nursing* (2nd ed.). Philadelphia, PA: F. A. Davis.

Gostin, L. (2008). *Public health law: Power, duty, restraint* (2nd ed.). Los Angeles, CA: University of California Press.

Grad, F. (2004). *The public health law manual* (4th ed.). Washington, DC: American Public Health Association.

Longest, B. (2005). *Health policymaking in the United States* (4th ed.). Washington, DC: Association of University Programs in Health Administration.

Policy Formulation and Implementation

Policy formulation and implementation are stages of the policymaking process that occur after much political activity that ensures that a policy issue arrives on the policy action agenda. Policy formulation and implementation stages continue to be impacted by political activities. The policy formulation and implementation stages of policymaking continue to be a transformative period of time in which policy continues to be influenced and defined. The context in which policy formulation occurs impacts the eventual policy that is formulated and implemented into practice.

Policy Development Context

Policy development is contextually dependent. The context in which policy development occurs includes the various policy agendas, political spheres, and interdependent discourse among various individuals and interest groups that represent scientific, social, and governmental interests. Constituents engaged in the policy development and formulation process negotiate with policymakers regarding the authorization and allocation of scarce resources while balancing the public's need against multiple other competing interests.

The various factors that influence the policy development context consists of public and societal need, special interest groups desires, political agendas, social and economic pressures, personal desires, and governmental influence. The context for policy development influences the political process, political maneuvers and strategies implemented, frames the policy issue, and impacts the resultant intent of the policy formulated. An aspect that influences the policy development context is the public's perspective.

Public Policy Perspective: Pluralist and Elitist

The public's perspective regarding the policy can influence the context in which the policy is developed. Two primary public perspectives that influence policy development are pluralistic and elitist. The pluralist perspective embraces the idea of multiple special interests affecting the development of policy as a means of ensuring equal representation in the policymaking process. Pluralists support that competing special interest groups should engage in the policy development process. From the pluralist perspective, the various competing special interest groups are viewed as counterbalancing forces in the policy development process as a means to ensure that the ultimate policy developed presents the best interest of the public. Group theory provides a supporting theoretical foundation for the pluralist perspective. Truman (1993) summarizes the essential tenets of group theory politics as: (1) special interest groups are essential linkages between the people and the government; (2) interest groups compete with each other in the political process to create a counterbalance of special interest; (3) no special interest group is dominant; and (4) special interest group competition is fair (Longest 2005; Truman, 1993).

In contrast to the pluralist perspective, the elitist values the input of a select few individuals in the policy development process. The elitist considers special interest groups to be ineffective and powerless (Longest, 2005). For the elitist, the majority of the policy power structure lies in the hands of a few who are influential through the financial wealth. In addition, the elitist entity may be a small group of individuals who are most influential due to their personal or professional positioning among networks of policymakers or through their affiliations. These groups of individuals are frequently referred to as the "power elite." The power elite have a financial basis from which to directly or indirectly influence framing of policy issues and impact policy development. The central tenets of the power elitist theoretical basis are: (1) real power rests with a small proportion of the general population; (2) members of the power elite have similar values and interests; (3) incremental policy change is preferred over radical transformative change; and (3) the elitists ensure that policy does not erode their power bases (Dye, 2010; Porche, 2003). The elitist perspective has been characterized as primarily concerned with self-interest.

Policy Formulation

Policy formulation occurs within a context of high political diplomacy and negotiation. The policy formulation process is a dynamic and continuous process that occurs within a larger political arena. The manner in which policy is formulated is referred to as the policy formulation approach. These approaches are described below:

Policy Formulation Approaches

There are two general approaches to policy formulation. These two approaches are rational and incremental (Mason, Leavitt, & Chaffee, 2007). The type of policy approach informs and shapes the policy development process. In addition, the policy formulation approach impacts the sequence of activities that occur during the political process of policymaking.

The *rational* approach reflects "real-world" goals. In the rational approach, policymakers define the problem; identify and rank social values aligned with the policy goals; examine policy alternative solutions in relation to both the positive and negative consequences of each alternative; conduct a cost and benefit analysis; compare and contrast options; and finally, select the policy that achieves the resolution that most closely aligns with social values and meets the most needs (Mason, Leavitt, & Chaffee, 2007).

In the *incremental* approach, policymakers initiate small policy changes in an evolutionary manner over time. Most policymaking is incremental. The incremental approach begins with the current *status quo* and alters the current policy through a series of incremental changes in relation to the expressed desire. The incremental approach permits greater involvement and permeation over time of various political systems within the political arena. Both approaches to policy formulation are dependent on the policy agenda, political environment, and policy issue.

In contrast to these two approaches, another possible approach to policy formulation is transformational. A *transformational* approach to policy formulation is comprehensive in nature. Transformational policy formulation proposes wide-spread policy change to entire programs or systems at once. Even though the proposed changes in the form of policy occur at one point in time, the implementation of various aspects of the transformational policy change may occur over a period of time.

Policymakers in the Governmental Branches

The governance power structure in the United States is balanced through the development of three branches of government. These three branches of government are the executive, legislative, and judicial. Through this governmental structure, the main policymakers are executives or bureaucrats, legislators, and judiciary officials such as judges.

The policymakers in the executive branch primarily consist of presidents, governors, mayors, and city council officials. These executive branch officials prepare proposed legislation that may require legislative action. Frequently, the policymakers at the executive level can initiate immediate policy through the issuance of an executive order. In addition, these executive officials are responsible for the development of rules and regulations that "operationalize" the implementation of policy that was legislatively authorized. The executive agency officials, or bureaucrats, also collect, analyze, and transmit information that can influence the development of future policy (Longest, 2005).

Legislators are responsible to their voting public or constituency. Legislators are responsible for considering the pros and cons of each policy issue based on the public or their constituency's best interest. Legislators serve as the primary drafters of policy at the federal and state levels (Longest, 2005).

Judicial officials establish policy through the interpretation of laws, interpretation of federal and state constitutions, interpretation of rules and regulations of executive agencies, and the establishment of judicial procedures (Longest, 2005). In their role as interpreters, the judicial branch representatives also declare laws as constitutional or unconstitutional, which sets future precedent for policy development and formulation. Judicial officials interpret the intent and meaning of policy, which accordingly impacts the manner in which policy may be implemented (Longest, 2005).

Drafting Policy Proposals

Policy proposal ideas can originate from multiple sources. The executive branch of government is expected to initiate policy proposals that Congress can approve (Dye, 2010). In addition, "executive communication" from the executive branch influences or initiates policies that may be drafted by others outside of the executive branch. Members of the legislative branch also initiate policy proposals. In addition, citizens, organizations, and special interest groups can petition the government, through the First Amendment, to formulate policy. The proposed policy generated by these groups can be in the form of ideas, solutions, or drafted policy that may be introduced into the process by an elected official (Longest, 2005).

Legislative staff members are an influential group that directly and indirectly affects the drafting of policy proposals. Once a problem is on the policy agenda, elected officials frequently delegate proposal drafting to a member of their legislative staff team. In addition, legislative staff members are the gatekeepers that control access and the flow of information to elected officials. Therefore, legislative staff members indirectly control policy by controlling access to an elected official (Weissert & Weissert, 2000). Staff members frequently provide long-term consistency in an elected governmental office. Legislators and executive officers are elected and change office or may be subjected to term limits. Legislative staffers provide the historical and institutional memory helpful to newly elected officials. Frequently, legislative staff members orient the new legislator to current and critical policy issues, thus further shaping the elected official's policy agenda. As expected, this relationship between elected officials and the legislative staff is dependent upon trust. Other indirect influence on policy proposals by legislative staff occurs through the execution of their normal duties such as: research, scheduling, communicating with constituents, and writing draft policy proposals (Dye, 2010).

The drafting of policy proposals is the result of a team effort. Any member of the legislature or executive branch can draft a bill; however, only an elected official of the legislative branch of government can introduce a bill.

Once a legislator agrees to officially sponsor a bill, that legislator is responsible for the language of the bill.

Legislative Oversight of Policy

Bills introduced into the legislative process are numbered sequentially by date of introduction and referred to the appropriate standing committee. Each legislative committee has a specific scope of legislative authority. Bills that have broad focus may be referred to more than one standing committee for consideration and action. This type of legislative oversight occurs during policy formulation. Legislative oversight also occurs after a bill is signed into law.

Once a bill becomes law, the authorizing body frequently employs the evaluation process to determine the effectiveness of the law. This evaluation data is reported to the legislative oversight committee. The legislative oversight committee is responsible for monitoring the implementation and effectiveness of the policy as detailed in the law.

The most powerful source of legislative oversight occurs through the continual appropriation of funds for each respective law. The Legislative Reorganization Act of 1946 mandates oversight of laws by the legislative branch of government (Longest, 2005). This oversight is expected to achieve the following:

- Ensure adherence to the intent of the law
- Improve efficiency, effectiveness, and economy of governmental operations
- Assess the ability of the executive agency to manage and achieve the implementation of the law
- Ensure the implementation of policy in the public's best interest (Longest, 2005)

Nurses and Other Healthcare Professionals as Policymakers

Nurses and other healthcare professionals' discipline-specific knowledge and experience within the healthcare system provides them with a unique knowledge and experiential base from which to influence the development of policy. Nurses and other healthcare professionals can assume many roles in the policymaking process. The nurse or other healthcare professional as a scientist or researcher generates or validates the scientific basis that provides essential foundational evidence to support or refute various elements of the proposed policy. They can serve as members or organizers of special interest groups that focus on specific policy issues. These professionals can work with lobbyists or as lobbyists. Lobbying is the process used to influence policymakers through the political process. Nurses and other healthcare professionals have served as electioneers. Electioneering is the process of using personal and professional networks to assist a political candidate to secure an elected office. Nurses and other healthcare professionals are cautioned to ensure that their engagement in electioneering is conducted as a private citizen and not representing their employer unless there is clear expressed permission. As electioneers, nurses and other healthcare professionals serve as a community mobilizers. They also engage directly with the legislative branch as advocates.

Nurses and other healthcare providers can participate as legislative advocates. Legislative advocacy is a process of collaborating with policymakers or policymaking bodies to gather support or influence the policy development process. The legislative advocacy process consists of: (1) marshaling allies, (2) coordinating organizational advocacy structure to promote communication and decision making among the marshaled allies, (3) developing or partnering with coalitions, (4) collecting evidence and data regarding the policy issue, (5) defining and piloting the policy message, (6) revising the message and developing a communication or social media network, (7) cultivating relationships with the media to promote communication, and (8) diffusing the message into the public and political structures that have the ability to influence the policy (Porche, 2003).

Nurses and other healthcare professionals provide expert testimony regarding policy issues. Nurses and other healthcare providers, have many personal and professional experiences that reinforce relevance to the policy issue. These providers can also serve as experts and provide expert opinion testimony that substantiates a position supported by scientific evidence and professional experience. In addition, nurses and healthcare professionals are members of the public. Therefore, they can provide personal testimony that adds a personal dimension to policy issues that impact the public and healthcare systems. Personal testimony provides a first-hand account of the impact of policy on the individual.

Policy Models

Policy models provide a framework that specifies the processes through which policy evolves, develops, and emerges as a solution to a policy issue or problem. There are multiple models that provide frameworks that can be utilized to understand the policymaking process, intervene in the policymaking process, analyze policy, evaluate policy, and develop other strategies to politically influence future policy models.

Kingdon's Policy Stream Model

The Kingdon policy stream model describes the policy development process as occurring through three streams: problem, policy, and political. These three streams might be envisioned as free-floating, waiting for a "window of opportunity," to open for policy development. The window of opportunity is an alignment of the three streams into an environment that is considered prime for policy development.

The problem stream is the problem that is identified within the policy agenda. The problem stream poses a challenge for policymakers to focus on the problem and to provide a policy solution. The policy stream consists of the potential policy alternatives that can be developed and implemented to resolve the problem. The goals and ideas of the policy also constitute the policy stream. In addition, policymakers such as legislative staff, researchers, congressional members, and special interest groups are a part of the policy stream. In the policy stream, Kingdon envisions policies as free-floating, in search of a problem or person who is ready to assume the policy development challenge to link that policy with a problem. The political stream characterizes the persons involved in politics and the political environment that influence the policy agenda. When at least two of the three streams align, the context is primed, and the window of opportunity is considered open for policy development. Kingdon's policy stream model is also used to analyze policy. The streams framework provides the primary three elements—problem, policy options, and politics—from which to analyze policy development and implementation (Kingdon, 1995).

Stage-Sequential Model

Stage-sequential is a systems model that identifies sequential stages for the policy development process. The stage-sequential model consists of four stages: policy agenda setting, policy formulation, program implementation, and policy evaluation (Mason, Leavitt, & Chaffee, 2007).

The first stage is policy agenda setting. The identification and distinction of an issue vs a problem determines it's placement within the policy agenda. This identification of a problem that needs a resolving policy initiates the policy agenda-setting stage. The identified problem is framed into a policy concern. The policy agenda-setting stage attempts to place the issue or problem on the policy agenda for action. Placement on the policy agenda can assume one of three levels of consideration: discussion, action, or decision. The discussion agenda merely places the issue or problem within the policymaker's scope of attention. The action agenda signifies that the problem is moving through to the policy formulation phase. The decision agenda denotes the last phase of stage one. The decision agenda legitimizes the problem that will be confronted by policymakers during the legislative or regulatory process (Mason, Leavitt, & Chaffee, 2007).

Policy formulation represents the second sequential stage. Policy formulation consists of collecting information on the issue or problem, analyzing the information, disseminating the information to various constituencies, and drafting legislation. All interested stakeholders and constituency groups should be engaged in the provision of valuable information to inform the policy formulation process.

Stage three focuses on program implementation. In the program implementation stage, the executive agency or body charged with, or authorized to, develop the program or implement the policy must begin to draft guidelines, rules, or regulations to operationalize the policy. Proposed drafts of the guidelines, rules, or regulations are generally published in a public medium to provide the general public with an opportunity for comment. Typical publications are the Federal Register, State Register, or an official publication of the appropriate regulatory agency.

Program evaluation constitutes the last sequential stage. The program evaluation stage attempts to answer the question, "Did the policy effectively achieve what it was formulated to achieve?" The program evaluation stage determines the extent to which a program has accomplished the intended goals and objectives as designed by the policymakers. The ultimate question to be answered during this stage is "Did the policy resolve the problem?" In addition to evaluating the outcome of the policy, the process of implementing the policy is also evaluated and reported to the responsible authorizing body (Mason, Leavitt, & Chaffee, 2007; Porche, 2003).

Richmond-Kotelchuck Model

The Richmond-Kotelchuck model was developed to support prevention policies in the public health arena. The model identifies three essential elements for prevention: knowledge base, political will, and social strategy. All three of these elements are considered essential for prevention policy development to occur (Atwood, Colditz, & Kawachi, 1997).

The knowledge base in this model represents the scientific and administrative evidence used to make informed policy decisions (Richmond & Kotelchuck, 1991). This knowledge base is the area of concentration for research and analysis by public health professionals. This in-depth involvement is critical to the development of a scientific base with which to influence public health prevention policy.

Political will is society's desire and commitment to develop and fiscally support new programs, and provide or modify the existing support to established programs in alignment with the knowledge base and social strategies. Political will is dependent on a group's ability to influence policymakers such as politicians, legislators, stakeholders, and special interest groups. The scientific knowledge base influences political will and vice versa (Richmond & Kotelchuck, 1991).

Social strategy is the use of the scientific knowledge base and the political will environment to develop public health prevention policy. The social strategy capitalizes on existing social networks and relationships to initiate and improve desired programs (Atwood, Colditz, & Kawachi, 1997).

Local Public Health Policy Model

An example of a local public health policy model, described by Upshaw and Okun (2002), was used to influence livestock operations that impacted the public's health. This model consists of five major processes that facilitate the formulation of public health policy: preparing to act; clarifying the role and approach; involving the community; communicating the rule and rationale; and adopting, implementing, and evaluating the rule.

Executive Orders

An executive order is a legally binding directive issued by the chief officer of the executive branch of government at the national, state, or local level. Executive orders are a type of legal policy and can be issued by a president, governor, or mayor. Executive orders generally deal with domestic issues. Executive orders do not require congressional or legislative approval to take effect; the officer who issues the order determines the effective date. To ensure a balance of power, as required by our Constitution, Congress or most state legislative bodies can overturn an executive order with a two-thirds majority vote.

Incremental Policy Formulation

Incremental policy formulation or policymaking describes a slow evolution of policy. Incremental policy formulation may occur when there is not enough political support to ensure that a transformational policy change will be approved by policymakers. Incremental policymaking can use existing policies as a foundation from which to expand the original intent of a policy. The long-term goal, a desired new policy, is hoped to be achieved over time, and often employs utilization of the media to frame policy, and prime policymakers and constituents. This process represents small successive changes to an existing policy so that over time, the entire intent of the policy has been transformed.

Incremental policymaking is a considered a conservative policymaking approach. The incremental approach to policymaking allows policymakers to avoid political struggles that require extensive justification for new policy. However, incremental policymaking has been considered a disjointed approach to policymaking, that yields confusing and contradictory policies. Adhering to a comprehensive strategic plan will prevent disjointed policymaking when using this incremental approach. An incremental policymaking plan should include:

- A comprehensive policymaking goal that describes the desired policy intent
- An agenda-setting plan that describes what policies will be developed and a timeline for placement on the action policy agenda
- Identified policy modifications with a timeline for policymaking
- Development of a long-term political strategy for each policy modification that will occur over time
- Development of policy evaluation plans to provide data that support each successive policy modification

Policy Implementation Process

A critical element for effective policy implementation is the ability to develop systems in which there are clear and strong linkages between the constituent's goals, governmental goals, proposed policy, and planned activities or programs. Policy implementation refers to connecting the intention of the policy to the outcomes or results achieved from the policy (Smith & Larimer, 2009). Buse, Mays, and Waltz (2005) propose six necessary conditions for effective policy implementation. These are:

- Clear and logically established objectives that are consistent with a common goal
- Sufficient evidence to support a relationship between the proposed policy and the expected outcome
- Implementation process that facilitates compliance by implementers (incentives and sanctions)
- Committed administrative and legislative support for implementation
- Required resources are available
- Clear communication

- Support from the public, interest groups, and all branches of government
- Stable socioeconomic conditions

Similarly, from a statutory perspective, seven elements have been identified as critical to policy implementation. These seven elements are: clear goals; adequate causal theory linking the policy alternatives to the problem causes; adequate resources; hierarchical integration of executive agencies responsible for policy implementation; decision rules to guide the executive agencies implementation processes; commitment from the executive agency to implement policy in alignment with it's intent; and formal participation by constituents who support the policy objectives and who are impacted by the policy objectives (Smith & Larimer, 2009).

Once a bill is legislatively passed, the governmental executive officer must sign the proposed, thus making it a law. With the signing of a bill into law, the policymaking process moves from policy formulation to the policy implementation. This transition of the newly signed bill into law moves responsibility from the legislative branch to the executive branch (oversight evaluation responsibility may reside with a legislative standing committee). Policy implementation is a function of the executive branch of government.

The respective executive departments and agencies have oversight responsibility for the implementation of laws (Longest, 2005). Policy implementation consists of two cyclical processes: rule making and operation. Rule making and operation are two processes that are dictated by administrative law.

Promulgation of Rules and Regulations

Rule making is the establishment of formal rules and regulations necessary to fully operationalize the legislative intent of the law (Longest, 2005). Rule making is also known as the policy legitimization process. Policy legitimization is considered one of the final steps in the policymaking process. Policy legitimization occurs as a result of the open process of policymaking that permits the public to provide feedback on proposed rules and regulations through the promulgation of rules and regulation process (Dye, 2010).

The executive department or agency responsible for implementing the law must determine the intent and develop rules and regulations consistent with the legislative intent. The promulgation process requires the publication of the proposed rules and regulations for a specified period of time in the public domain to permit an opportunity for public input and comment. **Table 7-1** provides a summary of the rule-making process. The process for promulgating rules and regulations consists of:

- Publishing a "notice of proposed rule making" in the State Register or Federal Register, generally a draft of the proposed rules and regulations
- A public comment period that permits reaction and discussion of the proposed rules and regulations. Frequently, the executive department or agency may permit interested parties to submit a request for a public hearing on the proposed rules and regulations.
- Proposed rules and regulations are revised based on public comment and or hearings.
- Publishing of the wording of the final rule in the State Register or Federal Register
- Implementation of published rules (Longest, 2005)

Operation

After the rules and regulations have been promulgated, operationalization of the rules and regulations begins the operation process. Operation is the actual activity that occurs in carrying out the proposed law, such as conducting inspections, imposing fines, issuing permits, or starting new programs (Longest, 2005).

Diffusion of Innovation

Diffusion of innovation provides a theoretical framework in which to understand the dissemination and adoption of policy. According to Rogers

Table 7-1   Summary of Rule Making Steps

- Advanced notice of proposed rule making
- Notice of proposed rule making
- Notice of public hearing
- Notice of final rule
- Agency implementation and enforcement

(2003), an innovation can be anything that is perceived as new by an individual or group. An innovation can be an idea, practice, or resource (physical, human, or fiscal) that requires the acceptance and adoption by another individual or group. Therefore, an innovation can be a policy, or the implementation of a new program resulting from a policy. Diffusion represents the process by which an innovation is communicated through channels over time among members of a social system. This theoretical framework provides a means to understand this diffusion process and to impact the rate of diffusion.

There are four main elements that affect diffusion of innovations: innovation, communication channels, time, and the social system or contextual environment. Each of these elements has an essential part in the rate of diffusion or dissemination of a policy within a population. The characteristics of an innovation that impact the rate of diffusion or dissemination, and ultimately adoption, are dependent upon the innovation's relative advantage, compatibility, complexity, trialability, and observability. These are briefly described below:

- Relative advantage—degree to which an innovation is considered better than what it will supersede
- Compatibility—degree that an innovation is considered consistent with existing values, past experiences, norms, and existing policies
- Complexity—degree to which an innovation is considered easy to understand and use
- Trialability—degree to which an innovation can be trialed or piloted with the option of returning to prior state before innovation adoption
- Observability—degree to which innovation produces visible results

Communication is the process by which individuals create and transmit information from one individual to another to promote mutual understanding. The communication channel is the means by which this message is transmitted. Time impacts the diffusion process through the innovation-decision process: innovativeness and rate of adoption. This innovative-decision process is a cognitive process by which an individual or group assimilates the knowledge regarding the innovation to formulate an attitude toward the innovation and render a decision to adopt, reject, implement or merely confirm a decision. This innovation-decision process involves five steps: knowledge, persuasion, decision, implementation, and confirmation. The innovativeness is the readiness with which an individual or group is likely to adopt innovation as characterized by five adopter categories. These adopter categories are:

- Innovators—first individuals to adopt an innovation; may serve as a gatekeepers
- Early adopters—next level of individuals to adopt an innovation; rely on opinion leaders to influence their adoption of innovation; not much ahead of the average individual in adopting an innovation; respected by peers for discrete use of new ideas
- Early majority—adoption of innovation takes longer than innovators and early adopters; act with peer base; most common adopter category; deliberate for some time before adopting an innovation; will not be the first or last to adopt an innovation
- Late majority—respond to increasing network and peer pressure to adopt an innovation; approach innovations with skepticism and cautiousness; adopt an innovation after most members of social system have adopted
- Laggards—last persons to adopt an innovation; prefer the past as their point of reference; resistant to change; suspicious of innovation and change agents; must be certain an innovation will not fail before it is adopted

The rate of adoption is the relative speed with which an innovation is adopted among members of an entire social system. The social system is considered a system of interrelated members or units that can be comprised of individuals, groups, or organizations and institutions.

Policy Modification

Policy is never perfect. As societal demands and policy agenda changes, there may be need for modification of existing policy. In addition, mistakes of omission and commission inevitably occur during the policymaking process. Policies are modified as a means to limit any negative impact of existing policy while continuing to meet the legislative intent and the public's need. Policy modification may be the result of policy analysis or policy evaluation processes that identify need for change or alteration in the existing policy. Policy modification engages several stages of the policymaking process such as agenda setting, legislation development, and promulgation of rules and regulations, depending on the extent and type of policy modification needed. The modification can result in an alteration to the original law, an amendment to the existing law, or modification in the rules and regulations that implement the law within the respective executive department or agency.

Policy Modification versus Policy Change

Policy modification and policy change are terms frequently used interchangeably. Policy modification and policy change are two distinct types of policymaking activities. Policy modification alters an existing policy by either deleting aspects of the policy, modifying aspects of the policy, or extending the original policy. Policy modification is frequently used with incremental policymaking. In contrast, policy change alters the entire focus and intent of the original policy. Typically, the original policy is superseded by a new policy.

Policy Development: Expanding the Scope of Nursing Practice

At the state level, Boards of Nursing engage in the development, formulation and regulation of the nursing scope of practice in accordance with the statutory authority. As societal need dictates, Boards of Nursing engage in a process of policy development to meet these societal needs within the respective state's legal statutory policy governing the scope of nursing practice. Frequently, this requires the development and formulation of policy in the form of statues or rules and regulations that expand the existing scope of nursing practice.

The policy development process for Boards of Nursing to explore expansion of the nursing practice scope consists of the following:

- Examining the existence of statutory authority that permits the expansion of the nursing scope of practice
- Exploring the history of practice for nurses that will engage in the expanded scope
- Analyzing the requisite educational, training, and experiential requirements for the expanded scope of practice

- Critiquing and synthesizing literature (with a focus on empirical research) that supports the expanded scope of nursing practice
- Determining the presence of or need for regulations that support this expanded scope of nursing practice
- Documenting the verifiable need for nurses to engage in the expanded scope of nursing practice
- Analyzing the evidence that supports the expanded scope of practice in relation to the impact of societal need, public health and public safety

Each health professional discipline has a different regulatory process. Professional regulatory boards establish the guidelines and standards to govern the methods of expanding the respective disciplines scope of practice. The method of expanding scope of practice for nursing described above is similar to other health professional disciplines. The policy development process presented above should be used as a general framework to guide expanding scope of practice. Nurses and other healthcare professionals should refer to their respective state regulatory board to define the specific process for scope of practice expansion within the respective state.

Policy Termination

Policy Termination is an aspect of the policy process that is not frequently discussed, but should be provided the same emphasis as policy formulation and implementation. Policies that are inaccurately terminated can result in the development of other policy issues and problems. Frequently, policy termination results in the elimination of programs, fiscal retrenchments, and the redirection of or expansion of existing policies and/or programs. Policy termination could even result in the closure of departments, organizations, or agencies.

Policy termination can be complete or incremental. Complete policy termination ends the cumulative policy at one specific point in time. Complete policy termination can be used as a political strategy to catch opponents "off guard" and reduce the resistance to policy termination. However, there could be considerable negative political fallout from such a precipitous maneuver if it is done abruptly and without notification. In contrast, incremental policy termination results from a progressive and consistent elimination of certain

Table 7-2   Policy Termination Recommendations

- Information leaks regarding policy termination should be minimized until a comprehensive plan and justification are prepared and ready for dissemination.
- Once a plan is developed, make use of the media to prime and frame the policy termination.
- Enlarging the policy constituency builds a support base for the policy termination beyond the original policymakers and supporters.
- The policy analysis and policy evaluation should include a harm analysis from the perspectives of the policy beneficiaries, supporters, and opponents.
- Maximize on societal and ideological changes to formulate a new perspective regarding the policy.
- Consider an external agent as the policy terminator.
- Do not encroach on power prerogatives.
- Provide positive incentives for terminating the policy.
- Use political strategies to adopt another policy as a replacement to the terminated policy.
- Consider terminating only nonessential portions of a policy.

aspects of an existing policy. Incremental policy termination is frequently associated with programmatic phasing out. The slow reduction of programmatic or organizational budgets is a means of incrementally terminating an existing policy or program. This is sometimes referred to as "decrementalism" (Lester & Stewart, 2000). **Table 7-2** provides some policy termination recommendations.

Summary Points

- Policy development is contextually dependent.
- The context in which policy development occurs includes the various policy agendas, political spheres, and interdependent discourse among various individuals and interest groups that represent scientific, social, and governmental interests.
- The context for policy development influences the political process, political maneuvers and strategies implemented, frames the policy issue, and impacts the resultant intent of the policy formulated.
- The pluralist perspective embraces the idea of multiple special interests affecting the development of policy as a means of ensuring equal representation in the policymaking process.

- The elitist values the input of a select few individuals in the policy development process.
- Policy formulation occurs within a context of high political diplomacy and negotiation.
- In the rational approach, policymakers define the problem; identify and rank social values aligned with the policy goals; examine policy alternative solutions in relation to both the positive and negative consequences of each alternative; conduct a cost and benefit analysis; compare and contrast options; and finally, select the policy that achieves the resolution that most closely aligns with social values and meets the most needs.
- In the incremental approach, policymakers initiate small policy changes in an evolutionary manner over time.
- Legislators are responsible to their voting public or constituency.
- Judicial officials establish policy through the interpretation of laws, interpretation of federal and state constitutions, interpretation of rules and regulations of executive agencies, and the establishment of judicial procedures.
- An executive branch prepares proposed legislation for legislative action by Congress or similar body depending on the level of government.
- Citizens, organizations, and special interest groups can petition the government, through the First Amendment, to formulate policy.
- Legislative staff members are the gatekeepers that control access and the flow of information to elected officials.
- Legislative staff members orient the new legislator to current and critical policy issues, thus further shaping the elected official's policy agenda.
- Bills introduced into the legislative process are numbered sequentially by date of introduction and referred to the appropriate standing committee.
- Each legislative committee has a specific scope of legislative authority.
- The legislative oversight committee is responsible for monitoring the implementation and effectiveness of the policy as detailed in the law.
- The nurse scientist or researcher generates or validates the scientific basis that provides essential foundational evidence to support or refute various elements of the proposed policy.
- Policy models provide a framework that specifies the processes through which policy evolves, develops, and emerges as a solution to a policy issue or problem.

- The Kingdon policy stream model describes the policy development process as occurring through three streams: problem, policy, and political.
- The stage-sequential model consists of four stages: policy agenda setting, policy formulation, program implementation, and policy evaluation.
- The Richmond-Kotelchuck model of policy identifies three essential elements for prevention: knowledge base, political will, and social strategy.
- The five major processes of the local public health policy model are: preparing to act; clarifying the role and approach; involving the community; communicating the rule and rationale; and adopting, implementing, and evaluating the rule.
- An executive order is a legally binding directive issued by the chief officer of the executive branch of government at the national, state, or local level. Executive orders are a type of legal policy.
- Incremental policymaking can use existing policies as a foundation from which to expand the original intent of a policy.
- Adhering to a comprehensive strategic plan will prevent disjointed policymaking when using this incremental approach.
- Policy implementation refers to connecting the intention of the policy to the outcomes or results achieved from the policy.
- Rule making is the establishment of formal rules and regulations necessary to fully operationalize the legislative intent of the law.
- Operation is the actual activity that occurs in carrying out the proposed law, such as conducting inspections, imposing fines, issuing permits, or starting new programs.
- An innovation can be an idea, practice, or resource (physical, human, or fiscal) that requires the acceptance and adoption by another individual or group.
- Diffusion represents the process by which an innovation is communicated through channels over time among members of a social system.
- There are four main elements that affect diffusion of innovations: innovation, communication channels, time, and the social system or contextual environment.
- The characteristics of an innovation that impact the rate of diffusion or dissemination, and ultimately adoption, are dependent upon the innovation's relative advantage, compatibility, complexity, trialability, and observability.

- The innovativeness is the readiness with which an individual or group is likely to adopt innovation.
- Policies are modified as a means to limit any negative impact of existing policy while continuing to meet the legislative intent and the public's need.
- Policy modification and policy change are two distinct types of policy-making activities.
- Policy change alters the entire focus and intent of the original policy.
- Policy termination can be complete or incremental.

References

Atwood, K., Colditz, G., & Kawachi, I. (1997). From public health science to prevention policy: Placing science in its social and political contexts. *American Journal of Public Health*, 87(10), 1603–1605.

Buse, K., Mays, N., & Walt, G. (2007). *Making health policy*. Berkshire, England: Open University Press.

Dye, T. (2010). *Understanding public policy* (13th ed.). Upper Saddle River, NJ: Prentice Hall.

Kingdon, J. (1995). *Agendas, alternatives, and public policies* (2nd ed.). New York, NY: Longman.

Longest, B. (2005). *Health policymaking in the United States* (4th ed.). Washington, DC: Health Administration Press.

Mason, D., Leavitt, J., & Chaffee, M. (2007). *Policy and politics in nursing and health care* (5th ed.). St. Louis, MO: Saunders.

Porche, D. (2003). *Public & community health nursing: A population-based approach*. Thousand Oaks, CA: Sage.

Richmond, J. & Kotelchuck, M. (1991). Coordination and development of strategies and policy for public health promotion in the United States. In W. Holland & R. Detels (Eds.), *Oxford textbook of public health*, (pp. 441–445). Oxford, England: Oxford Medical.

Rogers, E. (2003). *Diffusions of innovation* (5th ed.). New York, NY: Free Press.

Smith, K., & Larimer, C. (2009). *The public policy theory primer*. Boulder, CO: Westview Press.

Upshaw, V., & Okun, M. (2002). A model approach for developing effective local public health policies: A North Carolina county responds to large-scale hog production. *Journal of Public Health Management Practice*, 8(5), 44–54.

Weissert, C., & Weissert, G. (2000). State legislative staff influence in health policy making. *Journal of Health Politics, Policy and Law*, 25(6), 1121–1148.

Policy Analysis

8

Policies that have been formulated and implemented must be continually analyzed for currency with the political climate and social issues. Policy analysis provides valuable data that can assist with policy modifications. Policy formulation and modification is not the end of the policymaking process. Policies should be continually analyzed during all phases of the policymaking process, including agenda setting, policy formulation, policy drafting, rule making, policy implementation, and policy modification. Policy analysis is a strategy used to identify current policy issues and to assist in constructing policy formulation and modification strategies. Policy analysis also provides a perspective into the world of politics (Dye, 2010; Longest, 2005).

Policy analysis critically appraises the context in which an agenda issue or policy exists. Policy analysis is initiated with an interpretive analysis of the policy and a review of the historical evolutionary context of the policy. This policy analysis process may generate information regarding congruence between the present policy, and past and present political and social contexts. If there is significant incongruity in the policy analysis results, the analysis may initiate an in-depth policy evaluation; or the analysis alone could lead to policy modification recommendations. The product of policy analysis is a clear description of the problem, identification of policy solutions or alternatives, courses of action with expected outcomes, and a contextual understanding of the policy problem and comprehensive understanding of the policy.

Policy analysis can be conducted on three levels. Hudson and Lowe (2004) propose that macro-, meso- or micro-level policy analysis can be utilized. Macro-level analysis encompasses the broad parameters that influence policy such as global economics and globalization. Meso-level analysis focuses on the policymaking process through implementation and the individuals and groups that develop the policy. Therefore, the meso-level focuses on policymaking and policy implementation. Micro-level policy analysis focuses on the engagement between consumers or constituents and policymaking agencies or individuals and their personalities. The micro-level of policy analysis focuses on an individual's engagement, beliefs, and values that impact the policymaking process. In addition, the policy analysis model chosen will depend upon the intent of the analysis. Examples of different approaches are: examination of the specifics of the policy process (agenda setting, policy development, etc.); analysis of a substantive policy area (environmental health, smoking cessation, etc.); a prescriptive focus to determine what policy should be; or an empirical approach to existing policy. Therefore, prior to engaging in policy analysis, the analyst should define the level at which the policy will be analyzed and the overall purpose and intent of conducting the policy analysis.

Policy Analysis Models

There are two primary foci of policy analysis—analysis *of* policy or analysis *for* policy. Analysis *of* policy is a retrospective process that explores the determination of policy and what constituted the policy. Analysis of policy examines how policy evolved onto the policy agenda and the process of formulation of the policy. In contrast, analysis *for* policy is prospective and explores what may result if a respective policy is formulated and implemented (Buse, Mays, & Walt, 2005). Policy analysis is dependent upon access to data sources. Data sources used in policy analysis are outlined in **Table 8-1** An accurate policy analysis is dependent upon the use of valid and reliable documents. **Table 8-2** presents some questions to pose and consider when using documents as a data source in policy analysis.

Table 8-1   Policy Analysis Data Sources

- Policy documents
  - Legislation
  - Journals
  - Academic books
  - Position papers
  - Copies of public testimony
  - Annual organizational reports
  - Reports from think tanks, interest groups, consultants, governmental and nongovernmental agencies
- Interviews
- Focus groups
- Policy evaluation reports

Process Model

The process model identifies the stages of policymaking and then analyzes the determinants associated with each of the respective stages. In the process model, the policy analyst uses any policymaking model as the framework with which to conduct policy analysis (Lester & Stewart, 2000). **Figure 8-1** presents a conceptual policy analysis framework. The framework proposes the broad conceptual areas of content, process, actors, and context.

Table 8-2   Document Analysis

- Who authored the document? What are the author's political affiliations?
- Who published the document? What are their vested interest?
- What prompted the writing of the document?
- Does the document contain primary or secondary data sources? Is the document, in its entirety, a primary or secondary data source, or combined?
- What is the authenticity of the documents?
- How did the document frame the issue or problem?
- Is the document clear and logical?
- Can the document's contents be corroborated with other sources of data?
- Are there contradictory or competing interpretations of the document?

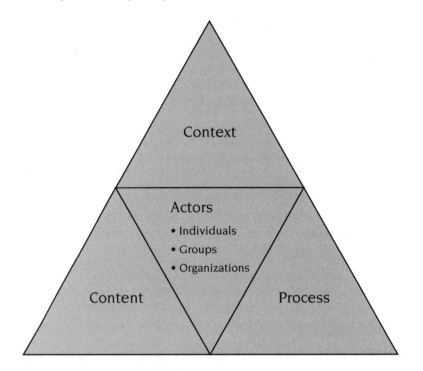

Figure 8-1   Policy analysis framework

Substantive Model

The substantive model analyzes the policy from the perspective of the policy issue. This analysis is usually conducted by policy content experts in the focus area. Policy analysts who engage in policy analysis using a substantive approach must not only be familiar with the content, but also with the political bodies and strategies used in policymaking in the focus area.

Eightfold Path

An eightfold path describes an iterative problem-solving process used to clarify the policy problem and determine policy solutions (Bardach, 2005). The eight iterative steps in this model are:

- Defining the problem
- Assembling the evidence
- Constructing policy alternatives

- Selecting the criteria
- Projecting the outcomes
- Confronting the trade-offs
- Deciding
- Telling the story

Defining the problem is the first critical step. The problem should be defined in quantifiable terms. These quantifiable terms permit the determination of the magnitude of a problem. In addition, the defining terms provide a baseline from which to evaluate the policy effect later. The defining of the problem permits the root causes of the problem to be determined. This differentiates the causes of the problem from the antecedent's associated factors, or consequences.

Assembling the evidence consists of collecting the data. Evidence assembly consists of reviewing the literature, conducting surveys to collect primary data, and synthesizing best practices. In the course of this process, people as a source of evidence will lead to other people, people will lead to pertinent documents, pertinent documents will lead to people, and documents will lead to other documents. Thus, evidence assembly is a tool that can provide cumulative evidence.

Constructing policy alternatives generates multiple policy options to resolve the problem or issue. It is from the policy alternatives generated that the final policy option is selected based on an evaluation of the appropriateness of the policy alternative to the problem.

Criteria selection determines the value system that will be used to evaluate the acceptability of a policy alternative. Typical selection criteria used are: efficiency in terms of cost-benefit analysis; justice (equality, equity, and fairness); freedom (free from government control, equality before law, free speech, religious freedom, privacy); legality; political acceptability; robustness and improvability; and linguistic clarity.

Outcome projection attempts to hypothesize the outcomes that will occur in relation to adoption and implementation of the policy alternative. Outcome projection also assists in identifiying unanticipated consequences that may occur.

Confronting the trade-offs is the decision process to determine the acceptable trade-off in positive and negative terms that will be permitted with the adoption of various policy options. The trade-off confrontation can be used to eliminate policy alternatives that do not meet the selection criteria and lead to more positive benefits.

Deciding and telling the story are the last two steps in the process. A final selection must be made from among the multiple policy alternatives. Telling the story consists of redefining the problem, reconceptualizing the policy alternatives, reconsidering the criteria, reassessing the outcomes, and reevaluating the trade-offs from the perspective that the selected policy alternative is the best. The storytelling must consider the audience, communication medium, and narrative story that connects the policy decision to the audience (Bardach, 2005).

Logical-Positivist Model

The logical-positivist model is also known as the behavioral or scientific approach. The logical-positivist model uses a deductive reasoning approach to policy analysis. The logical-positivist model begins with a theory or theoretical framework that guides the policy analysis inquiry process. The analyst then generates a model, and hypothesis testing examines the propositional relationships of the theoretical model. Data is collected and analyzed using either comparative or correlative measures, and findings are reported. This process is very similar to the research or scientific method process (Lester & Steward, 2000).

Participatory Policy Analysis (PPA)

Participatory policy analysis is a model that maximizes the democratic process. PPA uses a model that seeks input from participants to ensure that the ideals of a deliberative democracy are included in the generation of policy alternatives. This policy analysis model directly engages the constituents into the policymaking and analysis processes (Smith & Larimer, 2009).

Policy Analysis Process

The policy analysis process includes both intuitive and empiric components. Smith and Larimer (2009) describe the policy analysis process as an inquiry process that uses multiple methods of information gathering to produce policy-relevant information. The policy analysis process proposed by Smith and Larimer includes:

- Defining the problem
- Identifying the alternative policy course of actions
- Linking potential policies to outcomes
- Estimating the outcomes from each policy alternative
- Comparing the greatest impact and outcomes that will be generated among the various policy alternatives
- Selecting the most preferred policy alternative with the greatest potential impact and outcomes

A simple method for executing this process might be:

- Write down each potential policy decision or policy solution.
- Divide the paper in half under each potential policy decision or solution. Write the pros and cons for each policy decision or solution with the pros on one side and the cons on the other.
- Add a third column along with the pros and cons. In the third column, assign weights to each of the pros and cons reflecting the level of importance or desirability.
- Balance the pros and cons—strike out each pro and each con that cancel each other.
- Analyze the pros and cons to determine which side has the most weight.
- Use the final weights of the pros and cons of each policy solution to inform the decision-making process (Smith & Larimer, 2009).

The following framework has been described by Hewison (2007) as a foundation for a nurse manager's analysis of policy. The framework below was proposed for nursing but can be used to guide other healthcare professionals. The framework is:

- Identify the level of policy analysis: macro-, meso-, or micro-level;
- Use a nursing meta-paradigm to frame policy analysis that focuses on
  o Person (humanistic perspective)
  o Health
  o Environment
  o Nursing or other health professional discipline

- Examine the policy environment
  - o Understanding policy environment
  - o Response to organization's policy environment
  - o Manner in which organization's policy environment is shaped
- Develop an understanding of the manner in which the policy is developed
- Examine original sources of information generated during the policy development process to include parliamentary or legislative speeches, debates, committee minutes, official reports, government reports and documents, statistics, etc. Each policy document should be analyzed to:
  - o Develop a summary description of the main policy aims or objectives
  - o Establish the status of the policy document in comparison to other relevant documents
  - o Link policy document to other previous and associated policy documents
  - o Identify central policy themes or tenets
  - o Identify the area of practice impacted (can use nursing or the respective discipline's meta-paradigm)

Problem or Issue Analysis

An initial step in policy analysis is to analyze the problem or issue framing the need for policy development and formulation. Problem or issue analysis is a systematic process used to describe and explain the interrelationships of multiple antecedents or background variables affecting a societal concern (Porche, 2003).

A critical step in problem or issue analysis is distinguishing whether the area of concern is a real *problem* or merely an *issue* of concern. The ability to differentiate among problem situations, policy problems, and policy issues is critical to determining the most appropriate policy solutions. Problem or issue differentiation is dependent on stakeholders, constituencies, and policymakers' perceptions of the area of concern. A policy failure can be the result of inaccurately stating or characterizing the problem or issue. In addition, areas of policy concern that are *issues* can eventually evolve into what is considered a policy *problem*. The first step in discerning if the area of concern is a problem or issue is explore the areas placement within the policy agenda framework.

Issue Analysis Process

The differentiation of a problem and issue requires an analysis of the respective area of concern. This analysis is a 12-step process. During the analysis, debate and inquiry into the issue is encouraged, thus engendering insightfulness, inquisitiveness, and refusal to accept simple answers for complex queries (Porche, 2003). The following steps outline a process for the analysis of an area of concern and differentiation of the area as a problem or issue:

1. *Identification of the area of concern.* Identification of the area of concern clarifies the underlying and related concerns. Causes, potential effects, and interested parties are identified. The manner in which the area of concern may receive attention on the policy agenda is analyzed.
2. *Background.* The context of the concern is analyzed through an assessment of social, economic, ethical, political, and legal factors that are forcing the area of concern to rise to the level of the policy agenda.
3. *Stakeholders and constituents.* All direct and indirect stakeholders and constituents are identified.
4. *Position analysis.* Stakeholders' and governmental officials' (in the executive, legislative, and judicial branches of government as necessary) positions on the area of concern are analyzed.
5. *Political analysis.* The political climate is analyzed.
6. *Statement of concern.* A narrative statement is written delineating the boundaries of the concern. The concern statement may be altered throughout this analysis process.
7. *Interaction analysis.* The interrelationships of this area of concern with other issues or problems on the policy agenda are analyzed.
8. *Policy identification.* Potential policy options and alternatives are analyzed.
9. *Outcome identification.* Desired outcomes are identified.
10. *Policy recommendation.* The optimal policy solution for the area of concern is recommended.
11. *Impact assessment.* The depth and breadth of the area of concern is analyzed in terms of: the magnitude of this impact, the possible attachment of the concern to other policy issues and problems, political

context of the concern, and the potential for a finding of *issue* versus *problem*. A *problem* will have the greatest magnitude of potential impact, a network of attachment to other issues and problems, highly charged political attention, constituency and stakeholder readiness for action, and placement on the policy agenda for action.

12. *Determination.* The final labeling and framing of the area of concern as an issue or problem. This determination is contextual and changes as the policy agenda and political climate changes.

The final determination of whether the public health area of concern is an issue or problem is largely decided by interested parties and policymakers within the context of the area of concern. The magnitude of the concern frequently differentiates issue from problem. An area of concern considered a problem that needs policy intervention is frequently subjected to a detailed problem analysis. This process further structures the problem to facilitate policy development and formulation. There is some redundancy in the process of conducting an analysis of issues and problems, but this only leads to further clarification of the area of concern (Porche, 2003).

Problem Analysis Process

Problem identification consists of the following four steps: problem sensing, problem search, problem definition, and problem specification. Problem sensing is the recognition and felt existence of a problem. The problem sensing step analyzes the problem situation. The problem search step discovers the multiple representations of the problem, multiple stakeholders involved, and multiple worldviews of the problem. Problem definition formally characterizes the problem as a substantive problem. In the problem definition step, the problem is characterized in basic and general terms, and a conceptual framework of the problem is presented. The last step, problem specification, formalizes the problem through agenda setting, identifying constituents' needs, conducting public opinion polls, and assessing the opposition's position and strength in relation to the problem.

Several methods are used to structure or define a problem including the following:

- *Boundary analysis.* Identify the boundaries of the problem by posing the questions: What are the various facets of the problem? Who are the interested stakeholders and constituents? What are the multiple views regarding the problem?

- *Concept analysis.* Analyze the multiple concepts presented and discussed in the problem.
- *Hierarchy analysis.* Analyze the potential causes as possible, plausible, or actionable.
- *Synectics.* Analyze the similarities and differences of the problems.
- *Brainstorming.* Use this technique to generate goals, ideas, and policy strategies.
- *Multiple perspectives analysis.* Generate multiple explanations of the problem and potential policy strategies.
- *Assumption analysis.* Identify and synthesize multiple assumptions underlying problem and policy solutions.
- *Argumentation mapping.* Assess the accuracy of each assumption.

Problem structuring is critical to policy development and formulation. Problem structuring identifies the problem from the eye of the beholder, discovers and analyzes hidden assumptions about the problem, diagnoses possible causes, maps policy solutions, synthesizes conflicting views, and assists in designing new policy outcomes. The critical nature of problem structuring ensures that the correct problem is identified and that it is correctly characterized and solved through the development and formulation of the correct policy. The policy solution must match the problem.

A Summative Policy Analysis Process

Policy analysis is conducted on developed policy for a variety of reasons. Policy analysis facilitates a clearer understanding of the policy's intentions, expected outcomes, and interrelationships with other policies. Policy analysis is also conducted by regulatory agencies as a measure of rule making to implement required programs and to initiate policy modifications.

Policy analysis is a systematic process using methods that critically appraise the extent to which the policy is a viable and implementable solution to a problem and whether the policy will be acceptable to affected stakeholders and constituents given the current social fabric of society (Taub, 2002). There is a lack of consensus on the processes with which to structure the public health policy analysis process. Porche (2003) recommends the following process as one possible method of conducting policy analysis:

1. *Critical policy review.* The policy needs to be read repeatedly until there is clear understanding of the policy's intent and the various directives buried in the policy. The essential components of the policy should be outlined and correlated to current and past issues or problems. The policy should be reviewed for inconsistencies or gaps. The critical policy review should include an analysis of any components of the policy that appear to be unrelated amendments to the policy. The boundaries of the policy should be defined during this process. The policy boundaries inform the policy search process and parameters of the policy search.

2. *Policy search.* Conduct a comprehensive policy search that focuses on the problem. Policies that are affected by, or related to, the public health policy should also be analyzed. The related impact of one policy on another, or contradictions in two related policies should be assessed. Each of the related policies should undergo policy analysis.

3. *Historical analysis.* The time period in which the policy was developed should be reviewed in relation to social, economic, political, and environmental factors that influenced the policy. The values, beliefs, and political affiliations of the policymakers who drafted the policy at that time should be reviewed. Refer to Appendices A and B to determine the political context present during the respective time period at the national level.

4. *Authorization analysis.* Analyze the authorization legislation for the respective policy. Determine the scope of the authorization and the executive agency responsible for the implementation of the policy.

5. *Budgetary analysis.* Analyze the appropriation of funds to support the policy. Determine which components of the policy had the largest appropriation of resources. This provides some idea of legislative priorities in regard to the policy.

6. *Public health issue and problem analysis.* The issues surrounding the policy should be analyzed. The analysis should also address the problems identified in the policy as it currently exists.

7. *Stakeholder and constituency identification.* Actual or potential stakeholders, constituents, and special interest groups should be identified. The political positions of these groups regarding the problem and policy under review should be analyzed.

8. SWOT *analysis*. Identify the strengths, weaknesses, opportunities, and threats (SWOT) to the potential policy. The SWOT analysis should focus on the current analysis of the problem and the viability and adequacy of the existing policy to solve the problem.

9. *Gap analysis*. The provisions of the current policy in relation to the current needs should be appraised. Any gaps between the policy and the needs should be identified as potential areas for policy development, formulation, or modification.

10. *Executive summation*. A concluding brief summation of each of these steps should be developed and presented to policymakers. The final component of the executive summation should include recommendations for policy development, formulation, or modification. The final recommendations should include suggestions for authorization and allocation legislation. In addition, recommendations for the assignment of the implementation to the respective executive agency and the responsible legislative committee for the policy evaluation should be included.

11. *Prioritization*. Recommendations provided in the executive summation should be prioritized for policy development, formulation, modification, and implementation.

Summary Points

- Policy analysis provides valuable data that can assist with policy modifications.
- Policy formulation and modification is not the end of the policymaking process.
- Policy analysis is a strategy used to identify current policy issues and to assist in constructing policy formulation and modification strategies.
- The product of policy analysis is a clear description of the problem, identification of policy solutions or alternatives, courses of action with expected outcomes, and a contextual understanding of the policy problem and comprehensive understanding of the policy.
- Macro-, meso-, or micro-level policy analysis can be utilized.
- Analysis *of* policy is a retrospective process that explores the determination of policy and what constituted the policy.
- Analysis *for* policy is prospective and explores what may result if a respective policy is formulated and implemented.

- The substantive model analyzes the policy from the perspective of the policy issue.
- Eightfold path describes an iterative problem-solving process used to clarify the policy problem and determine policy solutions.
- Logical-positivist model uses a deductive reasoning approach to policy analysis.
- Participatory policy analysis (PPA) uses a model that seeks input from participants to ensure that the ideals of a deliberative democracy are included in the generation of policy alternatives.
- The policy analysis process is an inquiry process that uses multiple methods of information gathering to produce policy-relevant information.
- Problem or issue analysis is a systematic process used to describe and explain the interrelationships of multiple antecedents or background variables affecting a societal concern.
- A critical step in problem or issue analysis is distinguishing whether the area of concern is a real *problem* or merely an *issue* of concern.
- The final determination of whether the public health area of concern is an *issue* or *problem* is largely decided by interested parties and policy-makers within the context of the area of concern.
- Problem identification consists of the following four steps: problem sensing, problem search, problem definition, and problem specification.
- Problem structuring identifies the problem from the eye of the beholder, discovers and analyzes hidden assumptions about the problem, diagnoses possible causes, maps policy solutions, synthesizes conflicting views, and assists in designing new policy outcomes.
- Policy analysis is a systematic process using methods that critically appraise the extent to which the policy is a viable and implementable solution to a problem and whether the policy will be acceptable to affected stakeholders and constituents given the current social fabric of society.

References

Bardach, E. (2005). *A practical guide for policy analysis: The eightfold path to more effective problem solving.* Washington, DC: CQ Press.

Buse, K., Mays, N., & Walt, G. (2005). *Making health policy.* Berkshire, England: Open University Press.

Dye, T. (2010). *Understanding public policy* (13th ed.). Upper Saddle River, NJ: Prentice Hall.

Hewison, A. (2007). Policy analysis: A framework for nurse managers. *Journal of Nursing Management*, 15(7), 693–699.

Hudson, J., & Lowe, S. (2004). *Understanding the policy process: Analysing welfare policy and practice*. Bristol, UK: The Policy Press, University of Bristol.

Lester, J., & Stewart, J. (2000). *Public policy: An evolutionary approach*. Stamford, CT: Wadsworth/Thomson Learning.

Longest, B. (2005). *Health policymaking in the United States* (4th ed.). Washington, DC: Association of University Programs in Health Administration.

Porche, D. (2003). *Public & community health nursing practice: A population-based approach*. Thousand Oaks, CA: Sage Publications.

Smith, K., & Larimer, C. (2009). *The public policy theory primer*. Boulder, CO: Westview Press.

Taub, L. (2002). A policy analysis of access to health care inclusive of cost, quality, and scope of services. *Policy, Politics and Nursing Practice*, 3(2), 167–176.

Policy Research, Evaluation, and Quality Improvement

R esearch is the planned, systematic collection and analysis of data that answer relevant questions within the existing state of science. The research community consists of researchers–scientists, scholars, practitioners, academicians, students of various disciplines, and constituents. The research community has the ability to influence policymakers through several processes. The general processes in which a researcher can influence policymakers are documentation and dissemination of research findings, policy analysis, and prescription for the use of research findings through the communication of research implications.

Research is a tool that can be used to influence policy and policymakers. Research data can be used to influence the perceived impact of an issue and provide baseline data from which to evaluate policy impact and outcomes. Both quantitative and qualitative data can provide critical information to influence policymaking. Hanney, Gonzalez-Block, Buxton, and Kogan (2003) assert that research-informed policies are a secondary research output that can later be utilized as data for systematic review to inform future policy.

Policy Research

Policy research can be used to analyze a problem or as a means to further define the boundaries and context of an identified problem. Policy research is a tool to generate, gather, and disseminate information that informs the actions of policymakers. Weiss and Bucavalas (1980) propose four characteristics that define what is considered useful research by policymakers. These four characteristics are: research quality, conformity to expectations, action orientation, and challenge to the status quo. Therefore, policymakers are not just seeking solutions in policy research but also challenge the current political and policy paradigm. Six recommendations to increase policymakers' use of policy research are:

- Understand information needs.
- Understand the policymaking process.
- Target research findings to specific audiences and provide action-oriented policy recommendations from the research findings.
- Communicate research findings in understandable terms.
- Connect research findings to existing knowledge or expectations.
- Provide the context of the research findings and promote public debate of the findings.

In summary, policy research consists of study that relates to or promotes the public interest. Policy research is a broad term used to describe the comprehensive and systematic intellectual approach to the examination of problems.

Policy Research Process

The research process is a decision-making process based on the scientific process. The scientific process consists of posing a question, conducting background research on the subject area (reviewing literature), developing a hypothesis, testing the hypothesis, analyzing the data, drawing conclusions from the findings, and communicating the results. Fain (2004) proposes that the research process consists of five phases. The five phases are: selecting and defining the problem, selecting a research design, methods, data analysis, and research utilization. **Figure 9-1** outlines a summary of the phases of the research process.

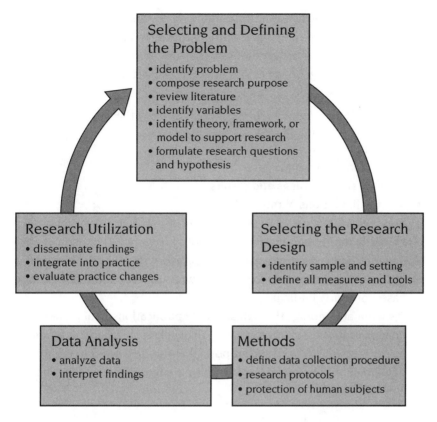

Figure 9-1   The research process

The policy research process integrates the research and policymaking processes (Wakefield, 2001). Policy research can be utilized to identify policy solutions or to generate knowledge in relation to information gaps regarding policy issues. Policy research involves quantitative, qualitative, and mixed-method research designs. The research design selected is determined by the policy research question posed and the knowledge gap. Some policy research may be evaluative type research of a program implemented from a policy, or action type research focusing on the behaviors of politics, policymakers, and individuals implementing the policy. The following process is suggested to facilitate the policy research process:

- Define the policy issue and the policy through a comprehensive review of the related relevant issues. The first step of a policy research project may be the conducting of an analysis of the existing or proposed policies.

- Conduct a review of scientific literature and statistical data.
- Develop research questions, study purpose, and hypotheses as appropriate. Some research variables to consider in policy research are information regarding: policy environment, policy action agenda, political actions and behaviors of policymakers and constituents and constituent groups, public opinion, and communication patterns.
- Select the research design.
- Select the research methods.
- Select data analysis methods.
- Propose study findings and results.
- Identify limitations of the study.
- Identify further recommendations to include practice implications, policy solutions, and future area of policy research. The research recommendations should be written to provide direction to policymakers regarding policy solutions or strategies to resolve the policy issue based on study findings.
- Disseminate findings through scholarly publications; oral presentations; distribution to appropriate policymakers, legislative bodies, and executive agencies; produce reports that can be posted in the public domain; inform media of findings; prepare testimonies on findings.

Research Utilization

Research utilization is a systematic process by which research data and knowledge formulated from research findings are integrated into practice (Fain, 2004). The practice arena includes but is not limited to the clinical practice environment. The practice arena includes the practice of developing and formulating policy, which is known as the practice of policymaking. The utilization of research is dependent upon the last stage of the research process, research dissemination. **Table 9-1** summarizes several research utilization models.

Research Utilization Models

Research utilization models provide a framework from which to incorporate the use of research findings into the policymaking process. Some framework models for research utilization are: the classic/purist/knowledge-driven model, problem-solving/engineering/policy-driven model, interactive/social

Table 9-1   Nursing Research Utilization Models

The following are some select nursing research utilization models. The process of each respective model is briefly summarized below:

Model	Process
Western Interstate Commission for Higher Education	• Problem identification • Research retrieval • Research review • Development of research-based care
Conduct and Utilization of Research in Nursing	• Problem identification • Assessment of knowledge base • Design of practice change • Clinical trial • Adoption or rejection of change • Diffusion of innovation into practice • Institutional change
The Nursing Child Assessment Satellite Training Project	• Recruitment • Translation of research findings • Dissemination of findings • Evaluation

interaction model, enlightenment/percolation/limestone model, political model, and tactical model. The classic/purist/knowledge-driven model uses a linear sequence of policymaking activities. In this model, research generates knowledge that then drives policymaking decisions. The problem-solving/engineering/policy-driven model also uses a linear sequence. It begins with problem identification by the constituent who requests the researcher to explore viable policy solutions. The researcher then explores various policy solutions and recommends the most appropriate policy solution based on research findings. The interactive/social interaction model closely resembles action research. This model proposes interactions between the researchers and users of the data to frame the research questions, and to process and use the research data based on the researcher's and user's needs. The enlightenment/percolation/limestone model proposes the use of research based on the gradual "sedimentation" of insight, theories, concepts, and perspectives. In the political model, politics influences all aspects of the research process from problem identification to research dissemination and implementation. Lastly, the tactical model uses research under the duress of pressure to act on an issue. In the tactical model, policymakers act by commissioning a study on the issue of concern. This is sometimes considered a political maneuver prior to engaging in the policymaking process.

Hanney, Gonzalez-Block, Buxton, and Kogan (2003) propose a model that places policymaking within the research utilization process. The model is described to exist within the context of the reservoir of knowledge and the political and professional environments of the wider society. The stages of the model are briefly described below:

- Stage 0—This stage initiates the research needs assessment. Stage 0 interfaces with Stage 1 with project specification, selection and commissioning.
- Stage I—This stage consists of the research inputs: prior knowledge gained form the needs assessment data and previous research findings.
- Stage II—Consists of the research process
- Stage III—This stage consists of the primary outputs from the research (data) that directly impacts the contextual knowledge reservoir that exists. This stage interfaces with Stage IV through the dissemination of the findings.
- Stage IV—This stage represents policymakers using the research data to inform policy and serves as a secondary output of the research,
- Stage V—This stage focuses on the application of research findings or utilization of research data in practice.
- Stage VI—This stage represents the cumulative final outcomes from the research that results from the implementation of the findings into practice and the resultant evaluation data, and the evaluation data from the implemented policy that resulted from the original research data findings.

Several nursing scientists have proposed models of research utilization that can be used in the policymaking process. These nursing research utilization models can be used by other healthcare professional disciplines engaged in the translation of science into clinical practice. Table 9-1 presented a summary of some nursing research utilization models. Regardless of the research utilization model implemented, the basic process of research utilization consists of:

- Problem identification, clarification, and refinement;
- Assembling the research literature;
- Critiquing the research findings;
- Synthesizing the research findings;
- Assessing the applicability of the synthesized findings;
- Implementing the research based innovation; and
- Evaluating the innovation (Fain, 2004).

Evidence-based Regulation

Evidence-based medicine or nursing practice expands the concept of research utilization. Research utilization focuses on integrating research findings into practice based on the findings from formal, systematic research investigations. In contrast, evidence-based medicine or nursing practice integrates research findings; but also integrates information from best practices, clinical expertise, patient values, and other sources of information (Melnyk & Fineout-Overholt, 2005). Research utilization is considered a narrower term than evidence-based practice (Spector, 2010). Evidence-based practice assists with closing the publication gap. The publication gap exists when researchers or experts have information and data to inform practice but have not disseminated the findings yet into literature retrievable by the public. Evidence-based practice uses hierarchies of evidence to evaluate the effectiveness of interventions and to determine the strength of evidence. The evidence hierarchies inform the appropriateness or readiness of the respective information for integration into practice. **Tables 9-2** and **9-3** outline types of evidence and some evidence-based practice hierarchies, respectively (Stetler et al., 1998). Spector (2010) outlines the following steps for evidence-based healthcare regulation policy as a means to inform policymaking:

- Question formulation—Convert the information needed regarding regulatory practice into an answerable question.
- Identify and collect evidence—Review the literature and collect other information and data relative to the proposed question.
- Appraise the evidence—Critically appraise all evidence and note the level of evidence using an evidence hierarchy.
- Process data—Extract data; synthesize findings from multiple data and information sources; and integrate findings into a recommendation.

Table 9-2   Types of Evidence

- Research-based data
- Opinion-based
- Expert panels
- Patient views
- Professional expertise and experience
- Quality improvement
- Infection control
- Financial data
- Process and outcome evaluation data
- Population and demographics (population science) data
- Morbidity and mortality statistics

- Disseminate findings—Report to a larger audience or constituency.
- Evaluate effectiveness and efficiency—Evaluate this evidence-based regulatory practice process from the stage of question formulation to disseminating findings.

Several frameworks or models exist to provide a process for evidence-based practice that can be used to determine the best policy solution based on the best evidence. **Table 9-4** summarizes several key evidence-based practice models (DiCenso, Guyatt, & Ciliska, 2005; Hughes, 2008; Melnyk &

Table 9-3   Evidence Hierarchies

American Association of Critical-Care Nurses
I   Manufacturers recommendation only
II   Theory-based without research data; recommendations of expert group only
III Laboratory data with no clinical data to support
IV   Limited clinical studies
V   Clinical studies in more than one population of patients or situations
VI   Clinical studies in a variety of populations and situations

Stetler Evidence Hierarchy
I   Meta-analysis of multiple controlled studies
II   Individual experimental study
III Quasi-experimental study
IV   Nonexperimental study (descriptive, qualitative, case studies, etc)
V   Systematically obtained verifiable quality improvement, program evaluation, or case report data
VI   Opinions of national experts, national expert panel discussions, regulatory, or legal opinions

---

Table 9-4   Evidence-Based Practice Frameworks–Models

ACE Star Model
- Knowledge discovery
- Evidence synthesis
- Translation into practice recommendations
- Implementation into practice
- Evaluation

Iowa Model
- Population or knowledge focused trigger
- Topic prioritized for organization relevance
- Assemble teams
- Assemble relevant research and literature
- Critique and synthesize research and literature for use in practice
- If there is insufficient data, conduct research study
- If there is sufficient data to implement practice change, pilot change and evaluate
- Used data from pilot evaluation or research study to institute change
- Evaluate outcomes
- Disseminate findings

Stetler Model
- Preparation
  - Identify, sort, and select relevant research evidence
  - Consider all influential factors
  - Affirm priorities
  - Define purpose of investigation
- Validation
  - Critique and synthesize information gather in preparation phase
- Comparative evaluation–decision making
  - Evaluate synthesized data according to fit of setting, feasibility, substantive evidence, current practice
  - Decide to use, not use, or consider use
- Translation–application
  - Decide to use now in practice
  - Consider use but conduct an evaluation of an implementation pilot
- Evaluation
  - Evaluate routine practice outcomes

Fineout-Overholt, 2005; Stetler et al., 1998; Stetler, 1994). Evidence-based practice models can be utilized to determine the best evidence to inform policy decisions and as a means to evaluate the impact and outcome of policy recommendations.

Legal Research Process

The legal research process provides the foundation for a lawsuit and provides valuable information that can inform policymaking. Legal nurse consultants, paralegal professionals, and attorneys perform legal research as a means to identify case law. In addition, legal research provides information regarding the assessment of liability, value of a case, and to evaluate opposing counsel's trial strategy.

The legal research process includes searching for relevant case law. Each case reviewed during the legal research process contains information regarding the case name, case citation (decision date, docket number, and court name), brief case summary, headnotes or subject notes, attorney names, judge names, and the text of the case opinion. In the process of searching for case law, it is critical that the legal research process explore if the case law remains viable. The research process should explore whether the existing case law has been overturned, remanded, or cited by more recent case law. The legal research process consists of exploring for relevant statues at the local, state, and federal level that may be relevant to the issue being investigated (Aiken, 2004).

The Internet as a Research Tool

The Internet serves as an excellent source of information without geographical boundaries. The Internet provides access to interlinked data without any hierarchical structure. The Internet provides access to valuable factual information mixed with misinformation. The utilization of the Internet as a research tool requires that the user discern quality information from misinformation. **Table 9-5** provides a list of criteria that can be used to evaluate Internet sites.

Policy Evaluation

Policy evaluation measures the overall effectiveness and extent to which a policy has achieved its objectives (Dye, 2010). Policy evaluation is a systematic, empirical assessment of the effects of ongoing policies and programs

Table 9-5   Internet Source Evaluation Criteria

- Website
  - ○ Title of website is consistent with URL address.
  - ○ The website domain is consistent with information presented (edu for education, com for company, gov for government, and org for an organization).
  - ○ Website has stable and active URLs for all links.
- Authorship
  - ○ The author is cited.
  - ○ The author's academic credentials, certifications and licenses, and organizational affiliations are noted.
  - ○ The author's contact information is provided.
  - ○ Author's curriculum vitae or resume is published.
  - ○ Author is known in the field.
  - ○ Author is referenced by another known author or respected professional in the field.
  - ○ Biographical information is present.
- Analog to Peer Review
  - ○ Links to webpage by professor or other recognized professional.
  - ○ Inclusion of webpage in college course readings.
  - ○ Links to webpage by another professional organization or society.
  - ○ Content is referenced by others in the field.
- Timeliness
  - ○ A copyright date is present.
  - ○ Revision dates are posted.
- Content
  - ○ Evidence of peer review.
  - ○ Content presents facts or opinions.
  - ○ Content has appropriate depth and breadth.
  - ○ Information consistent with other sources.
  - ○ Evidence of conflict of interest or bias not present.
  - ○ Document presents balanced perspective on the issue.
  - ○ Document contains a reference list or bibliography.
  - ○ Document meets requirement for scholarly publication.
  - ○ Information is adequately and appropriately referenced.
- Publishing Source
  - ○ Publisher's name and contact information provided.
  - ○ Can a webmaster be contacted?
  - ○ There is an official logo or watermark associated with publishing source.
  - ○ The publishing source is recognized.
  - ○ Is there a relationship between the author and publishing source? If so, what is the relationship?

developed from the policies (Nachmias, 1979; Porche, 2003). This evaluative process focuses on measuring the impact of a policy and the implementation of that policy as intended by the policymakers. Policy evaluation poses the questions "What have we done?" and "What was the impact and/or outcome?"

The effect of policy should be measured based on the intent of the policy and impact on the policy's target population. Dye (2010) suggests that evaluation of the policy should focus on its effects on real-world conditions. Real-world effects that should be measured in the evaluation process are (1) impact on the target problem, (2) impact on the targeted group, (3) impact on nontargeted groups (spillover effects), (4) impact on future and immediate conditions of the problem, (5) direct cost in terms of resources devoted, (6) indirect costs, and (7) net analysis of benefits to costs.

Sabatier (2007) proposes that policy evaluation criteria should consist of economic efficiency, equity through fiscal equivalence, redistribution equity, accountability, morality conformance, and adaptability. Economic efficiency is determined by the net benefits associated with the policy allocation or reallocation of resources. Fiscal equivalence is determined by equality between a constituent's contributions to an effort and their benefits derived from the result. Redistribution equity occurs when resources are redistributed to poorer constituents. Accountability represents a sense of responsibility to the constituents whose resources are used and whom the policy should impact. Morality conformance ensures that policies comply with the value system, beliefs, and ethical norms. Lastly, adaptability is the extent to which the policy can be applied to other populations and situations.

The evaluative responsibility for policy may be articulated in the policy. Several strategies are used to evaluate the effectiveness of policy. Dye (2010) identified the most common strategies for conducting a policy evaluation: (1) congressional or oversight committee hearings, (2) annual program reports to Congress or an oversight committee, (3) on-site visits, (4) tracking of program benchmarks, (5) comparison of program to some professional standard, and (6) ongoing evaluation of constituent complaints. In addition, the General Accounting Office (GAO) is an arm of Congress established in 1921 that maintains the authority to audit federally funded programs' operations and finances. The GAO submits its findings to Congress and other oversight committees as appropriate, as an evaluative measure of programs developed and implemented as a result of public health policy (Dye, 2010; Longest, 2005).

Public accountability requires a comprehensive evaluation of the impact of policies in terms of the intent and expected outcomes of the policy. Porche (2003) suggests the following process as a procedure to evaluate policies:

1. Conduct a public health policy analysis.
2. Identify the goals and objectives of the policy.
3. Identify public health data to measure the effectiveness of the public health policy.
4. Identify the articulated timelines in the public health policy.
5. Collect data on the chronological implementation of the policy.
6. Collect public health data indexes that measure the impact of the policy on the public's health.
7. Determine the extent to which the public health policy objectives have been met.
8. Identify intervening variables or circumstances that may have a negative impact on the maximum effectiveness of the public health policy.
9. Provide recommendations to improve the impact of the public health policy.
10. Disseminate findings to policy makers, stakeholders, and special interest groups.

Policy Evaluation Models and Process

Policy evaluation provides data that documents the influence of policies on policy issues and problems. In addition, policy evaluation provides data on program outcomes that resulted from the development and implementation of policies that authorized and allocated funds for programs. Decision-making processes and implementation strategies regarding current and future allocation of scarce resources use evaluation data. Three reasons to evaluate programs that are developed as a result of policies, are: to provide elected officials and policymakers with evaluation data to demonstrate program accomplishments and provide that the legislative mandates or administrative policy requirements have been met; guide program decision-making; and determine the level of improvements in health outcomes that are directly or indirectly linked to the program (Green and Kreuter, 1999).

Monitoring

Monitoring should be included as an essential element in the evaluation plan as it provides continual feedback about the policy. Monitoring is an ongoing measurement, providing information about the policy accomplishments and progress toward the preestablished policy goals, objectives and outcomes. Program monitoring is defined by Rossi et al. (1999) as "the systematic documentation of key aspects of program performance that are indicative of whether the program is functioning as intended or according to some appropriate standard" (p. 192). Program monitoring can include such variables as service utilization, program organization, and outcomes. Therefore, this definition regarding program monitoring can serve as the basis for a policy monitoring definition. The following policy monitoring definition is provided to guide policy monitoring activities. Policy monitoring is a systematic process of collecting data related to policy issues or policy that provides a concurrent analysis of the policy issue or policy in relation to the expected goals, objectives, or outcomes of the policy issue or policy (Porche, 2003).

Structure, Process, and Outcome

The structure, process, and outcome model of evaluation was proposed by Donabedian. Donabedian (1996) provided this evaluation framework based on his management perspective. Structure evaluation assesses the environment in which policy is developed and implemented, and includes measures such as organizational structure, resources and resource allocation, policy adherence, legal requirements, and management and staff qualifications. Process evaluation measures the extent to which the policy is implemented as planned. Outcome evaluation determines the extent to which the policy has achieved the expected goals and outcomes.

Formative versus Summative

Formative and summative evaluations differ based on the evaluation time period. Formative evaluation occurs at designated periods of time during the implementation of the policy. Formative evaluation data provide the foundation for the summative evaluation. In a program structure that has objectives that lead to the accomplishment of program goals, the objectives' evaluation at designated time periods may correlate with the formative evaluation process. Formative is sometimes referred to as the on-going periodic evaluation. In this same program structure, the summative evaluation occurs at the conclusion of a designated period of time in which specific goals should have been achieved. Summative evaluation data is used in the decision-making process to determine if the program goal and outcome was achieved. Summative evaluation is associated with the policy's long-term expectations (Porche, 2003).

Impact versus Outcomes

Impact evaluation measures the immediate results achieved from the intended policy. In contrast, outcome evaluation measures results that are achieved in relation to resolving the root cause or associated factors. For example, the impact may be the number of persons who receive a service resulting from the new program developed through the authorization policy. However, the outcome would be the extent to which the problem is resolved resulting from the new program. An exemplar for a policy to reduce the rate of human immunodeficiency virus (HIV) infection in a specific population would consist of the impact evaluation analyzing the results of the number of persons educated or number of condoms distributed depending on the program design. In contrast, the outcome evaluation would be an analysis of the reduction in the incidence of HIV infection in the specific population for which the program was developed.

Process versus Outcome

Process evaluation analyzes the extent to which the policy is implemented in the manner planned. In contrast, outcome evaluation analyzes the extent to which the policy solution has affected the problem. The outcome evaluation seeks to measure what a policy has actually achieved. In policy outcome evaluation, it is necessary to link outcomes directly to the various aspects of the policy. These associated or causal relationships strengthen the need for the evaluation data collected. Additionally, in policy outcome evaluation, there should be a discernment between the gross and net policy outcomes. The gross policy outcome consists of all the changes in the outcome variables observed when evaluating the policy. A formula for gross policy outcome measures is:

Gross outcome =
Effects of policy + Effects of extraneous variables to policy + Design effects

The net policy outcome consists of the changes in the outcome variables that can be reasonably attributed to the implementation of the policy with a clear associated or causal relationship. Net policy outcome measures are more difficult to ascertain.

Efficiency Analysis

Efficiency analysis involves an evaluation of the cost benefit and cost effectiveness of policies. Efficiency analysis provides critical data to policymakers regarding the allocation of scarce resources among the various policy initiatives. In a cost-benefit analysis, the policy outcomes are expressed in monetary terms as described previously. In a cost-effectiveness analysis, the policy outcomes are expressed in substantive terms. For example, a smoking cessation policy that focused on reducing the negative health impacts of smoking would have a cost-benefit analysis that examined the dollar savings from reduced medical care cost for smoking-related illnesses compared to the policy implementation cost. In comparison, a cost-effectiveness analysis of the same policy would estimate the dollars that have been expended to convert a smoker to a nonsmoker.

Utilization-Focused Evaluation

Utilization-focused evaluation's basic premise focuses on utility and actual use. The primary focus of utilization-focused evaluation is the intended use of the data to inform policy and policy issues for policymakers and constituents. The guiding principles of utilization-focused evaluation are systematic inquiry, competence, integrity and honesty, respect for people, and responsibility for the general and public welfare. Utilization-focused evaluation proposes a collaborative approach to policy evaluation based on several premises. Utilization-focused evaluation does not prescribe a specific model or process but actually proposes a framework or philosophical approach to policy evaluation. Some of the utilization-focused premises are:

- Intended use of data by policymakers and constituents is the driving force.
- The use of evaluation data is considered with the initial design of the evaluation plan.
- Personal factors, interest, and commitments impact use of data.
- Stakeholder analysis is critical.
- Useful evaluations are designed and adapted to certain situations.
- Stakeholders or users are engaged in the evaluation planning process.
- Evaluators should be active, reactive, and adaptive during the evaluation process (Fetterman, 1996; Porche, 2003).

Logic Evaluation Model

Logic models are utilized to link program inputs (resources) and activities to program outcomes. Logic models are a tool used to: (1) identify short-term, intermediate, and long-term program outcomes, (2) link program outcomes to each of the program activities, (3) select indicators, and (4) explain to decision makers the time necessary to achieve the respective long-term program outcomes.

The components of a logic model are inputs, activities, outputs, and outcomes (short-term, intermediate, and long-term). Inputs are the resources that are placed into a program such as staff, partnering organizations, equipment, materials, and direct and in-kind funding. Activities are the events that occur to implement the program. Outputs are the direct products of the program activities. The outcomes are the intended effects of the program. Short-term outcomes are the immediate effects of the program. Some typical short-term outcomes are knowledge, attitudes, and skills. Intermediate outcomes include changes in behavior, normative change and policy changes. Long-term outcomes are typically achieved after years of program implementation. Long-term outcomes are typically measured in changes in morbidity and mortality data. **Table 9-6** and **Figure 9-2** present a logic model template and a sample logic model.

Table 9-6   Logic Evaluation Model Template

Inputs	Activities	Outputs	Short-term outcomes	Intermediate outcomes	Long-term outcomes

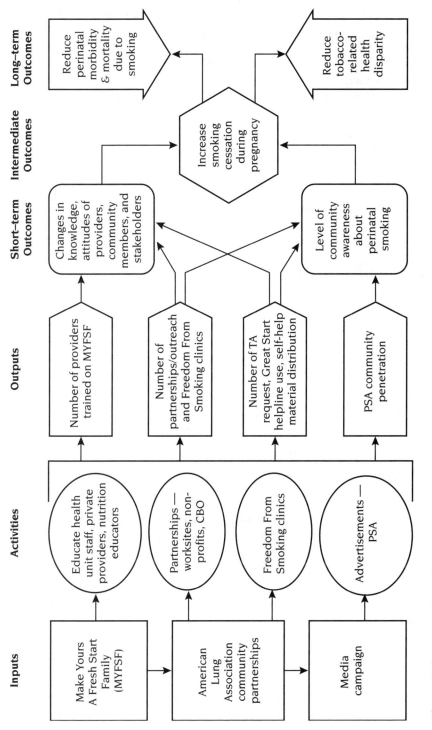

Figure 9-2   Perinatal smoking cessation program logic evaluation model

A logic evaluation model can be constructed with five steps. The five steps to constructing a logic evaluation model are:

- Step 1—Collect relevant background information regarding the policy or program.
- Step 2—Describe the policy problem and the contents of the policy or program.
- Step 3—Define the elements of the logic model—inputs, activities, outputs, short-term outcomes, intermediate outcomes, and long-term outcomes.
- Step 4—Draw the logic model in a figure.
- Step 5—Verify the logic model.

Research and Evaluation Informing Policy Formulation and Modification

Evaluation models and processes provide the guidance to ensure that the evaluation is correctly designed to generate the data and findings required to develop or modify existing policy. A sound policy evaluation must originate with a clear evaluation purpose and specific aims or objectives that guide the evaluation process. It is the evaluation questions, purpose and aims that direct the appropriate evaluation model and process to be implemented. Patton (1997) provides four criteria for evaluation models. These criteria are:

- Utilization—Evaluation provides valuable information to stakeholders.
- Feasibility—Evaluation is realistic, prudent, diplomatic, and frugal.
- Propriety—Evaluation is conducted in a legal and ethical manner with regard to the welfare of those involved and impacted.
- Accuracy—Evaluation process yields adequate and precise information.

Each evaluation model will utilize an evaluation design. **Table 9-7** provides a brief summary of evaluation designs. The evaluation design selected will depend on the evaluation question, purpose, aims, and evaluation model. A brief explanation of popular evaluation models and process are described below.

Multiple models and processes have been presented for the policy evaluation process. The following policy evaluation process is proposed as a means

Table 9-7   Evaluation Designs

- Experimental
  - Highest level of design.
  - Compares results between two or more groups.
  - True experimental studies have three required elements: manipulation of an independent variable, use of a control group, and randomization.
- Quasi-experimental
  - Resembles an experimental design with one of the required elements of an experimental design absent—frequently randomization is the missing member.
  - Used more for action research in natural settings.
- Mixed methods
  - Overarching evaluation purpose and aims require the collection of both quantitative and qualitative data.
- Nonexperimental
  - Common evaluation design
  - Nonexperimental designs can be descriptive, exploratory, comparative, or correlative in nature.
- Case study
  - An in-depth analysis of one specific case.
- Efficiency assessment
  - Measures cost effectiveness of policy implementation in relation to a monetary value.
  - Measures policy outcomes in reference to cost.
- Qualitative designs
  - Phenomenological
    - Examines the human-lived experience.
  - Ethnographic
    - Examines cultural issues.
  - Grounded theory
    - Focuses on the generation of a theory to explain a phenomenon.

---

to use evaluative data to inform the policy modification process. This proposed policy evaluation process is based on Porche's (2003) previous recommendations regarding an evaluation process for program evaluation and concepts presented in this chapter. The proposed policy evaluation process is:

- Engage policy and policy issue stakeholders, constituents, and policymakers.
- Define the purpose and objectives–aims of the policy evaluation.
- Describe the policy issue or problem.
- Describe existing policy, related or associated policies, previous policies, and policy alternatives.

- Design the evaluation plan.
- Collect evaluation data.
- Analyze evaluation data.
- Compose findings.
- Draw conclusions.
- Identify recommendations for practice, education, future research, and policy initiatives.
- Disseminate findings.

Policy Evaluation Dissemination

Dissemination should serve as the last phase of both the research and policy evaluation process. **Table 9-8** provides guidelines that promote the linking of the scholarly literature with policy.

Quality Improvement   .

Quality improvement data is another evidence source to provide input for policy development and modification. Quality improvement continually strives to move from a state of "good" to "great" while embracing change. The

Table 9-8   Guidelines for Linking Publications to Policy

- Explicitly link manuscript topic and title to policy.
- Frame the research findings or theoretical information within the current policy context.
- Background section of manuscript should reference and cite relevant policy.
- Manuscript should address populations of interest to policymakers.
- Language of manuscript should be understandable to policymakers.
- Manuscript should include policy-relevant content in the literature review and discussion sections.
- Manuscript should have information that can be used in multiple phases of the policymaking process.
- Manuscript content should be useful to political action committees, advocates, or special interest groups.
- Explicit policy terms should be used as keywords.
- Use current policy agenda terminology in manuscript and keywords.
- Manuscript should propose implications for policy in the conclusion.

focus of quality improvement is achieving quality. The structure, process, and outcome evaluation approach above is one approach suggested by Donabedian (1996) to improve quality. Deming (1982) identified fourteen points of quality. Deming's fourteen quality points are:

- Constancy—Create constancy of quality improvement purpose.
- Philosophy—Adopt a quality improvement philosophical perspective.
- Statistical data—Engage in data-based decision making.
- Price—Price cannot be the central focus when focusing on quality.
- Problem solving—Focus on problem identification and continually work to alleviate the problem or improve the problem level.
- Personnel training—Training is imperative to ensure quality.
- Supervision—Appropriate delegation with quality control measures in place
- Fear—Decrease fear inherent with making improvements.
- Barriers—Eliminate system barriers.
- Methods—Goals and methods are aligned
- Quotas—Eliminate quotas.
- Pride—Create a culture of pride.
- Education—The basis for knowledge
- Management—Top level and upper echelon support is critical to successful quality improvement efforts (Porche, 2003).

Quality improvement is one aspect of total quality management. Total quality management, as proposed by Deming (1986), consists of several basic principles. The basic principles of total quality management are customer focus, a continuous quality improvement obsession, continual improvement systems, unity of purpose, teamwork, employee involvement in the entire process, education and training regarding quality and quality improvement, a scientific approach, and a long-term commitment to quality (Porche, 2003). In addition, total quality management is based on the trilogy of quality proposed by Joseph Juran. The trilogy consists of quality planning, quality control, and quality improvement as interrelated processes (Juran & Godfrey, 1998). Quality planning consists of identifying customers, identifying customer needs, product development to address needs, establishing quality goals, developing processes to achieve quality goals, and improving process capability to achieve quality goals. Quality control consists of selecting the aspects of the policy, service delivery, or product development to control through a continual analysis of measuring specific quality indicators. Quality improvement consists of establishing the need for improvement, identifying projects for improvement, organizing the quality improvement project, conducting causal analysis for quality defects, identifying causes, implementing corrective action, evaluating corrective action plans, and providing controls to ensure integration of correction actions for continual improvement in the policy quality.

PDCA Quality Improvement

PDCA is a common quality improvement model. PDCA stands for plan, do, check, and act. The PDCA cycle consists of the following processes:

- Identify customers and policy stakeholders.
- Implement PDCA cycle
  - Plan—Plan the improved service.
  - Do—Implement quality improvements.
  - Check—Determine results and evaluate quality improvements.
  - Act—Integrate improvements into systems to maintain quality.
  - Analyze—Measure long-term quality outcomes resulting from improvements (Porche, 2003).

Summary Points

- Research is the planned, systematic collection and analysis of data that answer relevant questions within the existing state of science.
- The research community consists of researchers–scientists, scholars, practitioners, academicians, students of various disciplines, and constituents.
- Research is a tool that can be used to influence policy and policymakers.
- Policy research can be used to analyze a problem or as a means to further define the boundaries and context of an identified problem.
- Policy research is a tool to generate, gather, and disseminate information that informs the actions of policymakers.
- The scientific process consists of posing a question, conducting background research on the subject area (reviewing literature), developing a hypothesis, testing the hypothesis, analyzing the data, drawing conclusions from the findings, and communicating the results.

- Policy research involves quantitative, qualitative, and mixed-method research designs.
- Research utilization is a systematic process by which research data and knowledge formulated from research findings are integrated into practice.
- Research utilization focuses on integrating research findings into practice based on the findings from formal, systematic research investigations.
- Evidence-based practice uses hierarchies of evidence to evaluate the effectiveness of interventions and to determine the strength of evidence.
- The legal research process provides the foundation for a lawsuit and provides valuable information that can inform policymaking.
- The research process should explore whether the existing case law has been overturned, remanded, or cited by more recent case law.
- The legal research process consists of exploring for relevant statues at the local, state, and federal level that may be relevant to the issue being investigated.
- Policy evaluation measures the overall effectiveness and extent to which a policy has achieved its objectives.
- Policy evaluation poses the questions "What have we done?" and "What was the impact and/or outcome?"
- Policy evaluation provides data on program outcomes that resulted from the development and implementation of policies that authorized and allocated funds for programs.
- Monitoring is an ongoing measurement, providing information about the policy accomplishments and progress toward the preestablished policy goals, objectives and outcomes.
- Policy monitoring is a systematic process of collecting data related to policy issues or policy that provides a concurrent analysis of the policy issue or policy in relation to the expected goals, objectives, or outcomes of the policy issue or policy.
- Structure evaluation assesses the environment in which policy is developed and implemented; process evaluation measures the extent to which the policy is implemented as planned; and outcome evaluation determines the extent to which the policy has achieved the expected goals and outcomes.
- Formative evaluation occurs at designated periods of time during the implementation of the policy.

- Summative evaluation occurs at the conclusion of a designated period of time in which specific goals should have been achieved.
- Impact evaluation measures the immediate results achieved from the intended policy.
- Outcome evaluation measures results that are achieved in relation to resolving the root cause or associated factors.
- Process evaluation analyzes the extent to which the policy is implemented in the manner planned.
- Efficiency analysis involves an evaluation of the cost benefit and cost effectiveness of policies.
- The guiding principles of utilization-focused evaluation are systematic inquiry, competence, integrity and honesty, respect for people, and responsibility for the general and public welfare.
- Logic models are utilized to link program inputs (resources) and activities to program outcomes.
- The components of a logic model are inputs, activities, outputs, and outcomes (short-term, intermediate, and long-term).
- PDCA stands for plan, do, check, and act.

References

Aiken, T. D. (2004). *Legal, ethical, and political issues in nursing* (2nd ed.). Philadelphia, PA: F. A. Davis.

Deming, E. (1982). *Quality, productivity, and competitive position.* Cambridge, MA: Massachusetts Institute of Technology.

Deming, E. (1986). *Out of the crisis.* Cambridge, MA: Massachusetts Institute of Technology.

DiCenso, A., Guyatt, R., & Ciliska, D. (2005). *Evidence-based nursing:* A *guide to clinical practice.* Elsevier Mosby: St. Louis, MO.

Donabedian, A. (1996). Evaluating the quality of medical care. *Milbank Quarterly,* 44,166–204.

Dye, T. (2010). *Understanding public policy.* (13th ed.) Upper Saddle River, NJ: Prentice Hall.

Fain, J. (2004). *Reading, understanding, and applying nursing research* (2nd ed.). Philadelphia, PA: F. A. Davis.

Fetterman, D., Kaftarian, S., & Wandersman, A. (1996). *Empowerment evaluation: Knowledge and tools for self-assessment and accountability.* Thousand Oaks, CA: Sage.

Green, L., & Kreuter, M. (1999). *Health promotion planning: An educational and ecological approach* (3rd ed.). London, UK: Mayfield.

Hanney, S., Gonzalez-Block, M., Buxton, M., & Kogan, M. (2003). The utilization of health research in policy-making: Concepts, examples and methods of assessment. *Health Research Policy and Systems*, 1(2),1–28.

Hughes, R. (2008). *Patient safety and quality: An evidence-based handbook for nurses.* Washington, DC: Agency for Healthcare Research & Quality.

Juran, J., & Godfrey, A. (1998). *Juran's quality handbook* (5th ed.). New York, NY: McGraw-Hill Professional.

Longest, B. (2005). *Health policymaking in the United States* (4th ed.). Washington, DC: Association of University Programs in Health Administration.

Melnyk, B., & Fineout-Overholt, E. (2005). *Evidence-based practice in nursing and healthcare.* Philadelphia, PA: Lippincott Williams & Wilkins.

Nachmias, D. (1979). *Public policy evaluation.* New York, NY: St. Martin's.

Patton, M. (1997). *Utilization-focused evaluation: The new century text* (3rd ed.). Thousand Oaks, CA: Sage.

Porche, D. (2003). *Public and community health nursing: A population-based approach.* Thousand Oaks, CA: Sage.

Rossi, P., Freeman, H., & Lipsey, M. (1999). *Evaluation: A systematic approach* (6th ed.). Thousand Oaks, CA: Sage.

Sabatier, P. (2007). *Theories of the policy process* (2nd ed.). Boulder, CO: Westview Press.

Spector, N. (2010). Evidence-based nursing regulation: A challenge for regulators. *Journal of Nursing Regulation*, 1(1), 30–36.

Stetler, C., Brunnell, M., Giuliano, K., Morsi, D., Prince, L., & Newell-Stokes, V. (1998). Evidence-based practice and the role of nursing leadership. *Journal of Nursing Administration*, 28(7/8), 45–53.

Stetler, C. (1994). Refinement of the Stetler/Marram model for application of research findings into practice. *Nursing Outlook*, 42, 15–25.

Wakefield, M. (2001). Linking health policy to nursing and health care scholarship: Points to consider. *Nursing Outlook*, 49(4), 204–205.

Weiss, C., & Bucavalas, M. (1980). *Social science research and decision-making.* New York, NY: Columbia University Press.

Politics: Theory and Practice

P olitics is an integral aspect of the policymaking process. The majority of the population engages in political activities on a daily basis. However, politics is discussed and referred to as something that is negative and should not occur. This is much to the contrary. Political activity is a means to influence policymaking. What is not considered a positive aspect of influencing policymaking is illegal or unethical activities that may occur during political activities. This chapter provides a foundation to guide a professional's activities to influence the policymaking process.

Politics Defined

Politics is frequently associated with a negative connotation or belief system that encompasses something that is wrong. Politics also creates negative feelings and emotional responses such as anger, disgust, or indignation. In reality, politics and political maneuvers are a form of engagement universal to most interpersonal interactions. Politics is defined as the process of influencing someone or something to ensure the allocation of resources as desired. Politics and the political process use multiple forms of power. Politics is based on a power dynamic (Leavitt, 2009).

Ten Tenets of Politics

Political affairs involve the competing interests of individuals, groups, and sometimes societies or countries. The following ten tenets are provided to guide an individual's understanding of political environments as a means of promoting political power and political savvy. The ten tenets of politics are:

- Every vote counts.
- It all starts and ends at home, constituency is important.
- Know thy friends and enemies, keep both close enough to know their political agenda.
- The majority rules, always count your votes ahead of time.
- Build political capital, develop networks of influence.
- Politics involves economics, donate funds or generate funds.
- Exercise your power, negotiate for your agenda.
- Reputations are built over time, but destroyed in an instant.
- Politics is a personal sport, the best defense is a good offense.
- Exercise the 3 Ps—politeness, persistence, and persuasiveness.

Political Savvy and Astuteness

Political savvy and astuteness are competencies that increase an individual's ability to influence others. Political savvy is the knowledge, skill, intuitiveness, and perception regarding the politics of a given situation. Political savvy provides an individual with the ability to garner a clear perception of the political reality of a situation within a specific situational context, and recognize the impact of multiple alternative courses of action. Political savvy can be learned and developed with experience. **Table 10-1** presents strategies for cultivating legislative relationships. Political astuteness refers to an understanding of different political agendas and power bases among various individuals, organizations, and institutions and the dynamic between them in relation to the proposed policy solution. Some recommended strategies to increase political savvy and astuteness are:

- Learn the policymaking process and political strategies.
- Identify key individuals and constituents.
- Use networks to gain information and communicate.

Table 10-1   Cultivating Legislative Relationships

- Provide the legislator and staff with substantive information in a simple and comprehensive manner. Legislators like statistics and data.
- Be concise in your discussions.
- Be specific in your request.
- Provide public testimony if requested and as necessary.
- Consider compromise but know your limits of negotiation.
- Take notes during your meeting with the legislator or staff and follow-up with requested information or a note of thanks.
- Personal contact is preferred.
- Establish your constituency.
- Attend fundraisings.

- Participate in various levels of political engagement such as grassroots efforts, political action committees, or special interest groups.
- Increase your breadth of knowledge regarding current events by reading various newspapers of differing political opinions, books, and other publications.
- Listen to local, state, and national news programs.
- Serve on policy committees.
- Examine the local, national, or organizational culture and climate in relation to politics and the proposed policy.
- Understand the underlying social, political and historical factors shaping local and national political realities.
- Gain experience in a legislative or judicial office.
- Secure an appointed position as a board member.

Political Power

Political power encapsulates the total means, influences, pressures, and scope of authority used to achieve outcomes desired by the power holder. Political power is the ability to exert control over the behavior of another. Political power can be exerted with decision making and without decision making. Not making a political decision can be just as powerful as making a political decision. Political power can be considered potential or kinetic power. Potential power exists when an individual has the ability to influence another individual. This power may be present but is in a dormant state.

Table 10-2   General Political Strategies

- Persistence
- Incremental policy change
- Demonstration or pilot projects
- Frame the problem or policy within the context of known concerns.
- Be aware of covert messages, bring covert agendas into open
- Mobilize human capital and social networks.
- Quid pro quo—call in your favors
- Timing is critical—move when the window of opportunity exists.
- Exhibit a united front.
- Take measured risk.
- Use offensive strategies more than defensive strategies.
- Maximize your charisma.

Kinetic power occurs when an individual uses their power source to actually influence the behavior of another individual. **Table 10-2** presents general political strategies.

Two philosophical paradigms influence the means by which political power is used and cultivated. These are monolithic and pluralistic. The monolithic paradigm model is an authoritarian framework with a fixed power structure. In the monolithic paradigm, the authoritarian position at the top of the societal structure has the most power and exerts the most control. The monolithic paradigm embraces an elitist perspective in which the privileged minority rule. In contrast, the pluralistic paradigm embraces power from a grassroots perspective, which originates from the people. The pluralistic paradigm considers each individual, and multiple individuals forming social networks, as capable of exerting political power. The pluralist paradigm embraces open competition, freedom to organize into interest groups, openness to lobbying, the right to freely communicate views, and that no elite groups dominate (Buse, Mays, & Wilt, 2005).

The various stakeholders or constituents involved in policymaking processes have various levels and sources of power. The elements of power typically include instrumentalities (equipment, materials, funds), people, or information. The typical sources or types of power used to create political power include:

- Legitimate or structural —The authority associated with a specific position or role.

- Reward —The ability to provide incentives or rewards to another individual for a desired behavior.
- Coercive —The ability to exert a punishment on or by withholding something from another individual to achieve a desired behavior.
- Referent —The ability to influence others through associations with other individuals who have political power.
- Expert —The ability to influence others is a result of some specialized information or knowledge.
- Human resource —The ability to influence others resulting from interpersonal relationships or social networks.
- Material or resource —The influence exerted by controlling access to property, natural resources, or fiscal resources.
- Charisma or personal power —The ability to influence others based on certain attractive personal characteristics (Borkowski, 2005).

Political power is cultivated over time. Individuals who desire to influence policymaking should develop a political power base. The political power base can then be used at the appropriate time to influence specific policy outcomes. Several techniques to develop a political powerbase are:

- Cultivating social networks of persons who actively participate in policymaking, remain socially connected with individuals who engage in policymaking, or who control access to individuals engaged in policymaking
- Creating a sense of obligation so that an individual needs to return a favor
- Developing a reputation as an influential individual
- Developing a base of support
- Creating a favorable image within the public domain
- Public alignment with a problem or policy
- Creating a sense of perceived dependence among stakeholders
- Forming organized groups such as coalitions (Borkowski, 2005; Harrison & Shirom, 1999)

Iron Triangles

Members of an iron triangle are congressional members, members of the executive branch of government, and special interest groups. These three members form what is considered an unbreakable triad that proposes policy ideas and solutions. Some refer to the policy triangle as an iron clad issue network (Smith & Larimer, 2009). The iron triangle is a type of policy monopoly. Policy monopolies consist of structural arrangements that maintain the policymaking ability within a small group of interested individuals.

Through political affiliations, special interest groups coalesce together for a common interest and purpose. These groups frequently exhibit diverse types of political power throughout their vast networks. These groups that have and exert their political power to significantly influence policymaking are sometimes referred to as members of the "iron triangle." These iron triangles can consist of various constituents such as private interest groups, bureaucrats, and government officials who are linked together in mutually beneficial relationships. Members of the iron triangle are powerful fixtures within the policymaking arena.

Nurses' Stages of Political Engagement

Nurses should be politically involved in policy development, formulation, modification, analysis and evaluation. Nurses' engagement in the policy process has been shaped by educational preparation, practice experience, professional engagement, and the maturity level of the nursing profession. Cohen et al. (1996) identified four stages that characterize the political development of the nursing profession.

The first stage is considered to range from the 1970s to the 1980s. This stage is known as the "buy-in" stage. During this stage nurses were reactive. Their reactivity was characterized by the increase of nursing's political sensitivity. The second stage, termed the "self-interest" stage, occurred from the 1980s to the 1990s. During the self-interest stage nursing political engagement was characterized by the development of nursing's political voice. In the self-interest stage, nursing organized political action or special interest groups such as the American Nurses Association Political Action Committee. The third stage occurred during the 1990s. This stage is known as the "political sophistication" stage. In this stage, nurses began to be recognized as policymakers and healthcare leaders who had a valuable perspective and expertise in health policy. Lastly, stage four is known as the "leadership stage". This stage is characterized by nursing leadership in establishing policy agendas (Cohen, Mason, Kovner, Pulcini, & Scholaski, 1996; Mason, Leavitt, & Chaffee,

2006). Nursing is assuming leadership as a key interest group or stakeholder through organized political participation.

Political participation is one political engagement maneuver. Scholzman, Burns, and Verba (1994) define political participation as any formal or informal activity, that is mainstream or unconventional, and occurs as a result of individual or collective action to either directly or indirectly influence what the government does. Organized political participation is the engagement in activities of groups or associations whose political engagement is organized around specific goals and a policy agenda. Nurses' decisions to engage in political activities is influenced by resources, motivation, and engagement (Verba, Scholzman, & Brady, 1995).

Nurses must have the resources or wherewithal to engage in the political process. Resources identified to influence nurses' participation are free time, available money, and civic skills. The second influencing factor is the nurses' motivation to engage in political activity. Political interest, personal efficacy, and partisanship influence the nurse's motivation to engage in organized political activities. The last influencing factor is opportunity, or the network of recruitment that supports political engagement. These influencing factors consist of requests or cues to action that stimulate the nurse to become involved in an organization's political activities.

Organizational Politics

Organizational politics consist of the ability to influence another individual, group, or system within an organization. An individual, group, or systems can exert organizational politics. To effectively use organizational politics as a means of effecting policy changes, an individual must engage in the diagnosis of organizational politics.

Diagnosis of Organizational Politics

The purpose of diagnosing organizational politics is to gain an understanding of the political structure and forces that effect policymaking changes within a defined organization. The process of diagnosing organizational politics consists of three steps. The steps are stakeholder analysis, force field analysis, and identifying influencing tactics.

Stakeholder analysis consists of identifying the stakeholders with vested interest in the problem or proposed solution. The stakeholder analysis consists of examining each stakeholder's position, powerbase, and organizational role such as change agent, change strategist, implementor, policy recipient, or nonparticipating stakeholder. Each stakeholder's capacity for action in the policymaking process should be assessed along with the potential impact of their action.

The force field analysis maps the balance of forces for and against a proposed policy. The force field analysis identifies the restraining and supportive or driving political forces of change within an organization. The restraining forces strive to maintain the status quo. The supportive or driving political forces attempt to advance the political agenda toward a desired outcome.

Lastly, organizational politics diagnosis identifies the influencing tactics. The influencing tactics assess the tactical means used to influence others. The tactics could consist of, but are not limited to, framing or priming an issue, controlling access to powerful individuals, forming coalitions, and threatening the use of sanctions.

Table 10-3   Political Communication Strategies

- First impressions occur within the first 30 seconds.
  - Your first words should count.
  - Introduce yourself clearly.
  - Repeat the name of the person you meet.
  - Smile and face the person you meet.
- Work the room.
  - Survey the room.
  - Position yourself near a group to gain entry into their conversation.
  - Make eye contact to gain entry into a conversation.
  - Shake hands for the length of the introduction.
- Use humor cautiously.
- Speak with confidence.
- Be aware of nonverbal communication.
- Listen, do not speak over another person, and do not interrupt.
- Positive talk only, do not complain.
- Be culturally sensitive to interpersonal space.
- Exchange business cards with a note on the back to ensure you are remembered.

Communication: The Tool of Politics

Politics involves the ability to influence the allocation of resources. The tool used to influence individuals or groups is communication. Communication is the transfer of information from the sender to the receiver through a specific medium. In the policymaking arena, communication is not only the sending of information but is also used to receive information, educate, solicit feedback, and clarify meaning. **Table 10-3** presents some political communication strategies. **Tables 10-4, 10-5, 10-6, 10-7,** and **10-8** provide various samples of letters and guidelines that can be used in the political engagement of legislators.

Table 10-4   Congressional Letter Structure

Member of the House of Representative

The Honorable _____ (Name)
US House of Representatives
Physical Address
Washington, DC 20515

Dear Representative _____ (Name)*

[*If you are writing to the Representative in their capacity as a committee chair, the letter should be addressed as Chairman or Chairwoman. The Speaker of the House should be addressed as Dear Speaker _____ (Name).]

Member of the United States Senate

The Honorable _____ (Name)
US Senate
Physical Address
Washington, DC 20515

Dear Senator _____ (Name)*

[*If you are writing to the Senator in their capacity as a committee chair, the letter should be addressed as Chairman or Chairwoman. If the Senator is a majority or minority leader, the letter can be addressed as Dear Majority Leader _____ (Name) or Dear Minority Leader _____ (Name).]

Table 10-5　Guidelines for Policymaker Letters (Congressional or State Legislators)

Letters to policymakers should be to the point but persuasive. Consider the following guidelines in preparing a letter to a policy maker:

- Send the letter to the correct policymaker.
- Clearly and simply state purpose of letter.
- Focus on a single topic or issue.
- Letter should be unique and personal.
- Length of letter should be no more than two pages, preferably one page.
- Ensure a local perspective is presented.
- Inform the policymaker of your identity—who you are (establish constituency), and list your credentials.
- Provide factual information.
- Cite the specific bill number, proposed bill title, or name of act.
  - House bill: H.R. ____
  - House resolution: H.RES. ____
  - House joint resolution: H.J.RES. ____
  - Senate bill: S. ____
  - Senate resolution: S.RES. ____
  - Senate joint resolution: S.J.RES. ____
- Always close the letter with your requested action. Your request should be specific: "I request you to support/oppose ..." or "... vote for/vote against. ..."
- Use a professional and courteous tone.
- Close the letter with a reiteration of your specific request and provide all of your contact information.
- Proofread your letter for spelling, punctuation, grammar, and factual information.

Table 10-6　Sample Letter Format

The Honorable (First and Last Names)
Physical Address
United States House of Representatives
Washington, DC 20515

Dear Representative (Last Name),

I am writing to request your support/opposition to H.R. _____, _____ (Title of Bill or Act). This bill was introduced by Representative _____ on _____ (date). H.R. ____ and intends to _____ _____ (cite purpose of bill).

(continues)

Table 10-6   Sample Letter Format (*continued*)

[Next paragraph should focus on presenting your rationale for supporting or opposing the legislation. Ensure the presentation of facts and specific case information.]

[Concluding paragraph should iterate your request for support, or opposition to, the legislation (by specific number and name). Offer your assistance and provide your contact information.]

Respectfully submitted,

[Name, Credentials, Address]

Table 10-7   Sample Letter Format

The Honorable (First and Last Names)
Physical Address
United States House of Representatives
Washington, DC 20515

Dear Representative (Last Name),

As a constituent directly affected by (cite policy issue such as a disease, environmental issue, etc), I am requesting your support/opposition to H.R. ____ (number), _____ (name of bill). [Thank policymaker for past legislative support in related or similar issues that supports your current request.]

[Second paragraph can focus on providing statistical data, research information, and personal experience that provides background for your request.]

[Concluding paragraph should thank policymaker for their consideration. Cite your specific request again. Ensure that you request for authorization and allocation policy. Provide your contact information.]

Respectfully requested,

[Name, Credentials, Address]

Table 10-8   Sample Letter Format

The Honorable (First and Last Names)
Physical Address
United States House of Representatives
Washington, DC 20515

Dear Representative (Last Name),

As a voter and a constituent of _____ (cite city or county
and state), I urge you to support/oppose H.R. ___ (number), _____
(bill title). I also urge you to notify your colleagues in the House leadership,
_____ (list names) and in the Senate
_____ (list names) to inform them that you support/
oppose ____ (cite all bill numbers and titles related to the issue).

[Second paragraph should summarize your understanding of the intent of the
proposed legislation. Cite your specific data and examples to support your request.
You can also list your specific points of information you would like the policymaker
to consider, such as "I would appreciate your consideration of the following
informational points during your deliberation on ____" (cite issue—list the points,
logically, and succinctly).]

[Last paragraph should make one last profound and persuasive argument regarding
the impact of this proposed legislation. Cite your request one last time.]

Sincerely,

[Name, Credentials, Address]

Political Protocol

A political protocol consists of the written and unwritten rules that prescribe
the appropriate manner of engaging with political and elected officials during
formal functions and ceremonies. Political protocols exist to establish the order of precedence, rank, and power. Political protocol requires the utilization
of appropriate titles and forms of address, and proper etiquette for introduc-
tions and seating arrangements.

Political Theory and Philosophical Perspective Overview

Political theory provides the theoretical framework that identifies the essential concepts, assumptions, and propositions that describe, explain, and predict political action, political policies, and the exercise of political power (Heineman, 1996). Political theories can be systematic, ideological, empirical, or philosophical in nature. Systematic theories focus on the study of politics. Ideological theories focus on belief systems or the thought networks of political views. Empirical theories focus on quantitative data to describe, explain, and predict political behaviors. Lastly, the political philosophy theory places the study of politics within the larger nature of the universe and society.

Liberalism

Liberalism proposes an optimistic view based on the rational capability of individuals. Liberals believe in the ownership of private property and use of natural resources for individual human gain. Liberals emphasize support for democratic institutions, law, acceptance and tolerance of diversity, and peaceful reform (Heineman, 1996).

Socialism

Socialists are also referred to as Marxists. Socialism is monistic and materialistic. Socialism proposes shared property and wealth, and equal control and distribution of resources. Socialism focuses on the ability to produce product, or what is referred to as the forces of production. The material and systems used to produce the goods are owned by the state or country (Heineman, 1996).

Conservatism

Conservatives believes in the need to exert control and authority in society. The conservative perspective proposes that individuals with wealth and who are powerful in society have an obligation to provide resources and protect the less fortunate individuals in society. A conservative approach believes in a fundamental value system (Heineman, 1996).

Political System

A system is a complex whole that is greater than the sum of its parts. A system consists of a number of interrelated and interdependent parts or subsystems. Easton (1965) describes a political system as comprising inputs, through-puts (process), and outputs. The political inputs consist of the demands, resources, and support generated from the constituents. The demands on the system also result from the constituents' needs and desires. The inputs are placed into the system to generate policy outputs. The outputs are the public policies generated to provide goods or services that meet the constituents' expressed needs and desires. The process or throughput of the political system, consists of the policymaking process and political strategies that influence and impact the decision making that results in policy formulation.

Buse, Mays, and Waltz (2005) propose that political systems can be classified into five groups, based on the degree of openness to policy solutions and alternatives. These five groups are: liberal democratic regimes, egalitarian-authoritarian, traditional-inegalitarian, populist, and authoritarian-inegalitarian. The liberal democratic regime has stable political institutions that provide multiple opportunities to engage in political activities and strategies with a wide and diverse population representation. The egalitarian-authoritarian is similar to the elitist perspective—a few ruling elite individuals and an authoritarian autocratic bureaucracy. The traditional-inegalitarian rule through traditional monarchs which provides minimal opportunity for political participation in decision making. The populist system is based on single or dominant political parties. The authoritarian-inegalitarian is associated with military style governments that engage in repression as a form of political influence (Buse, Mays, & Waltz, 2005).

Similar to this classification, Heineman (1996) described three types of political systems: democratic, authoritarian, and totalitarian. The democratic system primarily exists in democratic societies. This system presents a political system in which political processes are decentralized and flexible. The democratic system uses interest groups, elections, and organized political parties as a means to influence policy. Authoritarian systems are characterized with strong centralized governmental control with strict limits on political activities. Free discussion, assembly, and association are limited in authoritarian systems. In the totalitarian system, propaganda is used to control the beliefs of the people and present a totalitarian and united front. In the totalitarian system, the government subordinates beliefs and behaviors to the needs of the government.

Political Process

The American democracy ensures a political process that provides each citizen with a voice. The political processes generally involve a multiparty political system. These political parties develop policy agendas and political platforms from which candidates generate their political campaign. Each candidate conducts a campaign to secure a nomination, or, for candidates who do not need a political party nomination, the campaign is used to promote their policy agenda or platform to persuade voters to support their candidacy. Constituents have an opportunity to engage in multiple aspects of the political process such as attending rallies, town hall meetings, listening to debates, reading about political candidates, campaigning, etc. Political strategies used in the political process are presented in a following section. **Table 10-9** provides some foundational terms inherent in the political process.

Table 10-9   Political Terms

Term	Brief Definition
Affidavit	A sworn statement in writing, usually under oath, or an affirmation before an authorized officer or notary.
Caucus	A meeting of a local party or organized group who engages in an open forum. Formal caucuses may engage in the selection of convention delegates to the party's national convention. In some aspects, caucuses may organize to inform members and debate policy issues.
Conservative	Emphasize free-market economic principles, prefer state and local government power over federal power, considered to be right of the center politically
Convention	A meeting at the state or national level that has delegates from a political party. Delegates cast votes to nominate individuals for political office.

(continues)

Table 10-9   Political Terms (*continued*)

Term	Brief Definition
Delegate	An official representative selected by members of their organization or party to represent the general membership.
Electoral base	A politician or political nominee's major constituency group that provides unprecedented support and loyalty to the candidate.
Electoral college	The electoral college is a group of popularly elected representatives who formally vote on behalf of the citizens for the president and vice president of the United States as mandated by the Constitution.
GOP	Abbreviated nickname for the Republican Party, stands for "Grand Old Party"
Independent	An individual voter who is registered to vote but has not declared an affiliation with a political party
Liberal	Individuals who are considered ideological, favor more power at the federal level and federal intervention into economic and social issues, considered to be left of the center of the political spectrum
Majority	A number greater than half of the total votes cast
Platform	A position or political agenda drafted by a candidate or political party to note their policy action agenda
Primary (closed or open)	A closed primary is an intraparty election open to only registered voters of the respective party. An open primary permits registered voters from other parties and independent registered votes to participate in the election.
Proxy	An individual authorized to act on another individuals behalf, generally a written document
Swing voters	Individuals who are not yet committed to a policy or politician's election, these individuals may still be persuaded to vote in a particular manner; also known as "undecideds"
Third party	A political party that exists outside of the Republican or Democratic parties

Voting

Voting is an American's ultimate voice in political policy, and is at the core of a democratic political process. Voting is a right that is exercised in the political process of elections. Elections involve four phases: voter registration, vote casting, collation and tabulation of votes, and certification of the results and announcement of the official results. The integrity of these three phases impacts the ultimate integrity of the political process.

As a truly democratic process, voting involves four critical properties—privacy, incoercibility, accuracy, and verifiability. Voters have the right to keep their ballots secret. Voters should not be unduly influenced in any manner. In the political process, integrity of the system requires accuracy in the final tally of the results. Lastly, verifiability ensures that voters can prove to themselves that they cast a vote as intended and the vote was counted.

Political Strategies

Political strategies are the methods and processes used to influence the desired policy goals. In addition to the general political strategies presented, specific political strategies include activities in, or use of: conflict resolution, lobbying, interest groups, advocacy, media, policy briefs, policy speeches, position papers, resolutions, and coalition building.

Conflict Resolution

The political process results in competing problems and policy agendas. The clash of competing interest may result in conflict. Conflict may be a direct or indirect result of the political process. Conflict is an incongruence in ideas, values, or beliefs between two or more individuals or groups. Conflict can result in antagonistic actions between two or more individuals or groups. There are four primary types of conflict—intrapersonal, interpersonal, intergroup, and organizational. Intrapersonal conflict occurs within an individual when there are conflicting values or opinions regarding the best policy alternatives. Interpersonal conflict occurs between two individuals. Intergroup conflict occurs between two or more groups. Organizational conflict can be a result of intrapersonal, interpersonal, or intergroup conflict that occurs within a defined organization. In addition to conflict resulting from incongruent ideas, values, or beliefs, conflict can be the result of disagreement regarding power and status.

Communication is the means of reducing conflict. Some communication strategies to resolve conflict are described in **Table 10-10**. Conflict resolution

Table 10-10   Conflict Resolution Communication Strategies

- Communicate and listen
- Clarify intent
- Clarify meaning
- Summarize discussion
- Paraphrase discussion
- Evaluate congruence between written, spoken, and nonverbal

is the process of resolving the incongruence into a mutually acceptable solution. Other conflict resolution strategies are:

- Denial or withdrawal—Avoids the conflict with the hope that it will resolve on its own
- Suppression—Downplays the magnitude of the disagreement
- Power or dominance—Resolves conflict through the use of positional power or authority, or majority rule.
- Compromise—Both sides forfeit something of value.
- Collaboration—Create a win-win situation in which both parties focus on a mutual goal.

Thomas and Kilmann (2002) propose that everyone has a preferred conflict resolution style. Thomas and Kilmann have developed a conflict instrument to measure an individual's conflict preference, know as the TKI, or Thomas-Kilmann Conflict Mode Instrument. The TKI identifies five conflict resolution modes that are used to resolve conflict:

- Avoiding—Do not address conflict, may withdraw or suppress feelings and actions
- Compromising—Identify a mutually acceptable solution that satisfies all parties involved.
- Accommodating—Neglect personal concerns to satisfy the concerns of the other party.
- Competing—Pursue own concerns at the expense of the other party.
- Collaborating—Mutually working together to explore an option that satisfies both parties (Thomas & Kilmann, 2002).

Lobbying

Lobbying is the process of approaching legislators or policymakers to present information to influence their decision making. Lobbying uses interpersonal relationships and power as a means of influencing decisions. The process of lobbying requires that the individual lobbying a legislator or policymaker to be informed on the policy issue or problem. In addition, the lobbyist must be knowledgeable regarding the legislative history of the issue, the power dynamics within the context of the issue, and the position of the respective constituents of the policy. **Table 10-11** presents lobbying tips.

Lobbying can occur through letter writing, personal visits, and email. Email provides an immediate mechanism to lobby a legislator. The following fundamental questions provide direction for lobbying interaction with a legislator or legislative staff regarding a policy:

- What is the proposed problem the legislation will resolve?
- What is the rationale for approaching the problem with this policy?
- Does a nonlegislative solution exist? What are the possible nonlegislative options?
- Has this policy or similar policies been proposed before? If so, what was the resolution?
- What is the fiscal impact of this policy?
- Who will sponsor the legislation?
- What special interest groups support, oppose, or remain neutral on the proposed policy? (Buppert, 2007; Ridenour & Harris, 2010).

Interest Groups

Interest groups are groups of individuals or organizations that share political, social, or other common interests, that seek to influence the policymaking

Table 10-11 Lobbying Tips

- Know the issue.
- Identify the communication medium, setting, time, and purpose of each lobbying interaction.
- Share an anecdote that illustrates the problem and policy resolution.
- Provide a fact sheet.
- Provide your business card with a special note on the back of the card.
- Provide any information promised, follow up within 1 week after the visit.
- Do not become argumentative.
- Request a statement about the position of the legislator on the issue and their voting intent.
- Conclude with a thank you note.

process. The benefits of interest groups are material, solidarity, and purposive. The material benefits exist from the sharing of tangible resources. The solidarity benefits include the power of masses or number of individuals. The purposive benefit includes ideological or issue-oriented goals. Buse, Mays, and Waltz (2005) propose the following seven functions of interest groups in our society—participation, representation, political education, motivation, mobilization, and monitoring of political behavior and policy.

There are different types of interest groups. Interest groups can be classified according to organizational structure, economic focus, benefits obtained, or goals and missions. Organizational structure designates the interest group as centralized or decentralized, or by level of focus such as local, state, or national. Economic interest groups focus on the economic interests of their constituents. Benefit interest groups seek to obtain some tangible deliverable for their constituents. Lastly, goals or mission interest groups pursue a common goal or purpose.

Lobbying is the primary activity of interest groups. Interest groups use either an inside or outside strategy for lobbying. The inside strategy is direct and focused in nature within the interest group. In comparison, the outside strategy focuses on influencing the general public external to the interest group.

Advocacy

Advocacy planning occurs after there is a determination for a need to change or propose a new policy. Advocacy planning is considered "a strategic planning process that specifies goals, an implementation strategy with key stakeholder analysis, a SWOT (strengths, weaknesses, opportunities, threats) analysis, timeline, budget, and evaluation plan" (Patterson, 2008, p. 778). Advocacy planning's impact is to inform the policy agenda, shape the policy agenda and inform policymakers regarding a specific policy solution. Patterson considers advocacy planning essential to ensure policy change occurs. The formula proposed by Patterson for policy change consists of:

Analysis + Advocacy Planning + Action = Policy Change

Political Action Groups

Political action groups or committees are frequently referred to as PACs. Political action groups or committees are the funding arm of special organizations or interest groups. These groups exert their political influence through financial contributions to a candidate's legislation or campaign. PACs use their constituents to raise funds to build their power base through the potential to make financial contributions. In addition, PACs engage in lobbying activities.

Media

The media has a critical role in policy agenda setting. The power of the media lies in the ability of editors, producers, anchors, reporters, and columnists to present policy problems or issues to the public within the public domain (Dye, 2010). The media exerts considerable influence in agenda setting. The media controls what is considered "news" and who is "newsworthy" (Dye, 2010). The media does not necessarily control what we think but they definitely influence what we think about.

Media influence occurs through two activities, priming and framing. Priming is the psychological process used to increase the salience of an issue through the activation of previously acquired information. Priming utilizes cognitive psychology theory. In priming, the media has the ability to plant an idea or concept within an individual's mind about a specific issue or related issue. This priming facilitates the manner in which an individual thinks about or judges future information regarding the issue. Priming sets the stage for future messages regarding a policy problem or issue (Domke, Shah, & Wackman, 1998).

Framing complements the priming process. Framing is the activity used by the media to focus our attention on specific aspects of an issue and obscuring the focus on other aspects of the issue (Prouty, 2000). Framing impacts the assimilation of information regarding a policy. The frames create the boundaries within which individuals think about the policy. Two primary forms of frames are episodic and thematic (Porche, 2003). Episodic frames focus on the current person in trouble or current point of conflict in relation to a problem or issue. In contrast, thematic frames focus on the context within which the issue is unfolding. The thematic frames place the problem, issue, or policy within a broader social, political, environmental, or economic context.

Both priming and framing influence thinking regarding policy problems and policy resolutions. Priming and framing can be utilized to secure support for a specific policy issue. Therefore, these are also considered policy interventions.

Media Analysis

Media analysis facilitates the assessment of the extent to which the information presented is biased or the manner in which the information is biased. Policymakers are advised to conduct a media analysis of several sources prior to formulating an opinion. A media analysis permits an individual to critically evaluate media messages, learn who controls the media, and determine vested interest that are projected into the information presented. A media analysis consists of examining: the medium of communication; who sends the message; what is the message delivered; the rhetoric used to convey the message; effectiveness of the message in influencing opinions, emotions and generating attention; and accuracy of the message. In addition to the use of media serving as a political strategy, responding to the media is also considered a political strategy. A typical response to the media might be an editorial or response to an editorial. **Table 10-12** presents some recommendations for writing an editorial.

Testimony

A testimony is an oral presentation delivered before a committee, organization, or an elected official. A testimony is typically an oral presentation of a position regarding a policy or policy issue. Oral testimony may be at the request or subpoena of a congressional or state legislative committee.

Table 10-12   Editorial Guidelines

- Opening paragraph
  - Outline the issue or problem.
  - Challenge an opinion or agree with an opinion.
  - Opening should be dramatic but factual.
- Second paragraph
  - Present your position.
  - Clearly state your rationale.
- Third paragraph
  - Acknowledge opposing thoughts or opinions.
  - Counter each opposing thought or opinion.
- Last paragraph
  - Present a call to action or challenge.
  - Be specific in your request for action.
- Signature—name, title, affiliation (if permitted), city, state

Table 10-13   Trial Testimony Guidelines

- Review all evidence and documents prior to the trial, especially your deposition.
- Wear professional attire.
- Convey confidence, sincerity, impartiality, and control.
- Speak clearly, keeping eye contact with the person asking the question, and as appropriate to the jury or judge.
- Provide succinct and precise answers.
- Answer only the question posed.
- Control your emotions and facial expressions.
- Remain within the limits of your knowledge, expertise, and credentials.
- Explain any terms that may be unfamiliar to the judge or jury.
- Do not discuss the case in public areas.
- Do not speak with any juror.

Oral testimonies may have severe time limitations, especially before congressional committees. It is imperative that the individual delivering an oral testimony secure the guidelines and procedures for the testimony prior to engaging in the delivery of the testimony. In the delivery of an oral testimony, adequate preparation is essential. The testifier must analyze the committee and their respective position on the policy or policy issue, research the policy or policy issue, and prepare the testimony with factual and experiential information. The oral testimony should be written so that copies can be submitted to the committee. This creates a public record of the testimony and serves as a resource for future reference. **Tables 10-13** and **10-14** present some guidelines for the delivery of an oral testimony (Kleinkauf, 1981).

Table 10-14   Legislative Testimony Guidelines

- Introduce yourself.
- Provide credentials.
- State who you are representing; it is critical to establish your constituency.
- Open with a position statement that clearly identifies the policy or issue to which you are speaking.
- Present the body of your speech using exemplars to connect with the committee and factual data to support your position.
- If speaking to a policy issue, ensure that you present your position relative to both sides of the issue with supporting evidence and exemplars.
- If presenting before a judicial committee, ensure that you discuss legal issues.
- Compare and align your testimony with other groups or organizations.

(continues)

Table 10-14   Legislative Testimony Guidelines (*continued*)

- Conclude with a specific request or call for action—be specific in what action you are requesting.
- Conclude by offering to answer questions.
- Avoid reading directly from a written testimony.
- Avoid shuffling papers.
- Make eye contact.
- Be aware of your voice projection and body language.
- Know the titles and positions of everyone on the committee.
- Address committee members by their official and honorary titles.
- Expect and be prepared to answer questions, do not become argumentative during the question and answer session. If you disagree, respectfully inform the person you disagree and present your position briefly.
- Follow-up is critical—always provide any information requested, and send thank you notes.

Policy Briefs

Policy briefs provide a quick explanation of the policy issue or problem and the proposed policy, along with policy and political assessments. The policy briefing provides a quick and informative snapshot of the issue and policy solution. Policy briefs can be written or oral. A written policy brief is frequently referred to as a "one pager." The typical policy briefing paper includes a summary of the issue, background information, policy alternatives, various stakeholder and constituency perspectives on each policy alternative, and recommended action. An oral policy briefing should be presented in a concise and logical manner that includes the same information described for a written policy briefing. **Table 10-15** presents the format for a policy brief (Jennings, 2002). **Table 10-16** presents guidelines that can be used to evaluate the quality of a policy brief (Britner & Alpert, 2005).

Policy Speeches

A policy speech intersects the principles of policymaking, politics, and public speaking. Policy speeches are conducted during political campaigns and during policy agenda setting and policymaking activities. Any individual who engages in public speaking to communicate a specific position regarding a policy can render policy speeches. **Table 10-17** presents some policy speech guidelines.

Table 10-15   Policy Brief Guidelines

- Introductory statement of issue
  - Clear statement of the issue or problem to be addressed
- Context and background of the issue
  - Most effectively written in bulleted format
  - Concise
  - Background of the issue
  - Key regulatory and legislative history
  - Provide data—statistics, demographics, recent trends
  - Current references for all data provided
- Policy options or alternatives
  - Present pros and cons of each policy option or alternative
  - Provide timetable for action
  - Present political perspective associated with each policy option and alternative
  - Present placement of each policy option within the policymakers policy agenda, values, and previous commitments
  - Present political vote count for each policy option if known
- Resources
  - Cite references

Table 10-16   Policy Brief Evaluation Criteria

- Quality of content
  - Cohesive and logical argument
  - Relevant research and data used
  - Integrated review of background information
  - Statements supported with references
  - Presents comprehensive perspective
- Organization
  - Clear statement of the issue or problem
  - Conclusions of current state of knowledge from convergent findings
  - Clear recommendations for action
- Quality of writing
  - Written at the appropriate level for the policymaker
  - Assumes no previous knowledge regarding subject matter
  - Objective and scientific
  - Appropriate use of grammar, spelling, punctuation
  - Concisely written

Table 10-17   Policy Speech Guidelines

- Introduction
  - ○ Establish credibility.
  - ○ Connect with the audience in opening remarks.
- Body
  - ○ Establish a slogan or memorable tag line.
  - ○ Describe the problem: give examples, connect with the constituents, give statistics.
  - ○ Present solutions.
  - ○ Illustrate the points.
  - ○ Use expert testimonials.
  - ○ Present advantages and disadvantages.
  - ○ Acknowledge other positions and render them nonviable.
  - ○ Present a call to action to your audience.
- Conclusions
  - ○ Review the problem.
  - ○ Restate the solutions and call to action.
  - ○ Conclude with a memorable closer.

Position Papers

A position paper is used to educate, generate support on an issue, and to formalize a position or agenda in relation to a policy issue. A position paper typically describes the individual's or organization's position on an issue, and a recommended solution with the supporting rationale for the position. The position paper is based on evidence with a sound argument provided. In addition, a position paper can introduce an organization's philosophical intent regarding a social or political issue.

A position paper is also known as a "white paper." The term white paper is used less often today to remain culturally sensitive to specific populations. The term white paper originated from the term white book, which was an official government publication. **Tables 10-18**, **Table 10-19**, and **Table 10-20** present position paper purpose, format, and guidelines.

Table 10-18   Position Paper Purpose

- Frame the policy discussion on the issue or problem.
- Organize and outline the position of an individual or organization.
- Formally inform other constituents about your position on the issue or problem.
- Present recommended policy solutions.
- Provide a framework from which to develop and formulate specific policies or resolutions.
- Establish a voice and credibility on the issue or problem.

Table 10-19   Position Paper Format

Organizations are encouraged to develop a consistent position paper template. In addition, organizations are encouraged to have a systematic process for the development and formulation of position papers, continual analysis and review of current and past position papers, method of archiving position papers, and process for the approval of position papers that includes a period of public or organizational comment and debate. If an organization is updating or developing a new position paper, the organization should identify previous or related position statements and clarify which position statement has supremacy or takes precedence. This can be accomplished through one statement "This position paper supersedes the position paper titled _____, ratified on _____ (date), by _____ (name of organization)."

Typical format of a position paper includes:
- Position paper should cite the mission of the organization, organizational identity, and organizational address, constituents represented
- Provide supporting evidence and data, factual information
- Consist of three sections of a position paper include
  - Introduction
  - Body
  - Conclusion
- Introduction
  - Identify the issue or topic of the position paper
  - A thesis statement that clearly presents the main idea of the position
- Body
  - Provide background information on the issue with supporting evidence and data.
  - Provide one idea per paragraph regarding the issue.
  - Build your argument logically with transition of thought between the paragraphs.
  - Provide a discussion of the supporting and opposing position of the argument. Clearly articulate your position and the rationale supporting your position.
  - Reference supporting organizations, legislation, regulations
  - Cite figures, tables
  - Provide cases or exemplars
  - Use primary source authoritative references, interviews, expert opinions, leader statements, indisputable dates or events
  - Body of the position paper should use an inductive logical reasoning approach
- Conclusion
  - Declaration of resolution to the issue
  - Suggest courses of action.
  - Reinforce ideas without repeating.

Table 10-20   Position Paper Guidelines

- Use official letterhead with organizational logo.
- Cite references.
- Provide contact information for leaders quoted.
- Paper should focus on a single issue or problem
- Thesis statement should articulate the main premise and position
- Both supporting and opposing arguments should be recognized.
- Provide rationale for the position.
- Length should be one to two pages
- An organizational position paper should include:
  - Brief introduction of your organization
  - Organizational history related to the issue, problem or topic
  - Impact of issue or problem on your organization
  - Organizational current policies with respect to the issue and supporting rationale for your policies
  - Quotes from your organizational leaders about the issue or problem
  - Statistics or empirical research that supports your organization's position
  - Actions taken by your organization related to the issue or problem
  - Past position papers or resolutions adopted and ratified by organization on the issue or problem
  - Organizational opinion or suggested resolution to the issue or problem

Resolutions

A resolution is a formal motion, position, or solution proposed by an executive or governing body or organization. A resolution consists of four parts: heading, subject, preamble, and operative clause. **Table 10-21** presents guidelines for writing each of the four parts of a resolution.

Coalition Building

A coalition is a group of individuals or group of organizations that form together around a common area of interest (Porche, 2003). Coalitions consolidate grassroots-level power and generate grassroots advocacy. Coalitions increase the political power structure by increasing the number of individuals supporting a specific policy. The power of coalitions is the ability to convene and bring together individuals from diverse perspectives, that focus on a clearly defined purpose, to achieve a common goal. Coalitions ensure a

Table 10-21   Resolution Writing Guidelines

- Format
  - Single spaced with double spacing between clauses
  - Each line should be numbered along the left margin of the paper
  - Each clause should begin with the appropriate introductory phrase
  - Preamble clauses end with a "," and the word "and"
  - The last preamble clause should end with a "."
  - Each operative clause ends with ";"
  - The last operative clause ends with a "."
- Resolution Heading
  - Provides the identification of the resolution
  - Where the resolution will be submitted
  - What is the topic
  - Who is the author
  - Sample heading:
    - SUBMITTED TO:
    - SUBJECT:
    - PROPOSED BY:
    - DATE:
- Preamble
  - First half of the resolution
  - Why the action of the operative clauses is needed
  - States any past action
  - First word of preamble clause sets the tone
  - Defines the purpose
  - Provides evidence and data to support the operative clauses
  - Initiating phrases for preamble clause

Acknowledging	Deeply disturbed	Observing
Affirming	Deploring	Noting
Alarmed	Desiring	Reaffirming
Anxious	Determined	Realizing
Appreciating	Emphasizing	Recalling
Approving	Encouraged	Recognizing
Aware	Endorsing	Referring
Bearing in mind	Expressing	Regretting
Being convinced	Expecting	Reiterating
Cognizant	Fulfilling	Seeking
Concerned	Fully	Stressing
Confident	Grieved	Welcoming
Conscious	Guided by	Taking into account
Contemplating	Having	Taking into
Convinced	Keep in mind	consideration
Declaring	Mindful	Taking note

(continues)

Table 10-21   Resolution Writing Guidelines (*continued*)

- Operative Clause
  - ○ Tells the reader the action needed
  - ○ First word should be a verb
  - ○ Initiating operative phrases:

Accepts	Deplores	Further resolves
Adopts	Designates	Instructs
Affirms	Directs	Reaffirms
Appeals	Expresses its	Recognizes
Appreciates	appreciation	Recommends
Approves	Expresses conviction	Regrets
Authorizes	Expresses its regret	Reiterates
Calls upon	Expresses sympathy	Renews its appeal
Commends	Expresses thanks	Repeats
Concurs	Expresses the belief	Suggests
Condemns	Expresses the hope	Supports
Confirms	Further invites	Takes note of
Congratulates	Further proclaims	Transmits
Considers	Further reminds	Urges
Decides	Further recommends	Welcomes
Declares	Further requests	

broad base of ideas, opinions, and expertise. In addition, each member or organizational partner of the coalition adds a different type of resource to the coalition. The cornerstones of an effective coalition are leadership, diverse membership, and diverse resource pool. The following are some suggested steps for the formation of a coalition:

- Define needs, objectives, cope of interest, and type of influence needed from coalition members.
- Analyze the breadth of influence of the coalition members.
- Secure resources needed to establish basic infrastructure of a coalition.
- Identify potential members of the coalition. This is an iterative process—as the coalition forms, and objectives are refined, the need for a specific type of coalition member will expand the search for other coalition members.
- Develop vision and mission statements.
- Convene public meetings of the coalition.

- Utilize feedback from coalition members to refine the vision, mission, and objectives of the coalition; invite more members; and develop strategic plans that include action work plans.
- Establish the coalition's identity (name, bylaws, logo, letterhead, brand identity, etc.).
- Develop coalition materials (fact sheets, position papers, policy briefs, etc.).
- Engage in advocacy or other defined activities of the coalition.

A goal of a coalition is to advance a specific policy agenda. The primary vehicles for advancing the coalition's agenda are communication and developing a financial base. Coalitions develop extensive networks through which to publicize their perspectives. The five Rs for effective advocacy are: having the Right preparation on the issue, using the Right communicator, sending the Right message, proposing the Right request, and Repeating the advocacy or lobbying efforts as necessary to ensure success (Berkowitz & Wolff, 2000).

Political Polls

Political polls are surveys used to measure the potential of a specific candidate to win an election or to determine the level of support for a specific issue or policy. Political poll results are a means to persuade individuals to the popular public opinion; however, political polls can be framed in a manner that demonstrates partisan support in a specific direction. Political polls are conducted in most elections. Exit polls are highly influenced by election turnout by constituents. Exit polls are expected to measure actual votes (Heineman, 1996). These exit political polls shape and form public opinion and sentiment as a means to prime and frame policy.

Public Opinion

Public opinion creates a "group think" mentality that may persuade some individuals to align their beliefs and actions with the majority, particularly if it is believed this will lead to a desired outcome. Public opinion informs and shapes policy agendas and potential policy alternatives. Public opinion is a good assessment of the national mood. Even though public opinion is a measure of the national mood, some problems with using this as a measure are that the public opinion or national mood may not reflect the public's true policy preference and that national mood is highly volatile with the ability to change without significant warning (Smith & Larimer, 2009).

Vetting

Vetting is a process of conducting a comprehensive background examination and evaluation of individual prior to appointing the person to a position or selecting the individual as a partner in a political campaign. Vetting can also occur before an individual is offered employment, especially for senior executive or upper echelon positions within an organization. The media engages in its own vetting process, typically within a public forum such as newspaper articles or televised news reports. The following steps are proposed as critical to ensuring a successful vetting process:

- Identify the characteristics needed for the respective position to include but not limited to knowledge, attitude, behaviors, skills, competencies, political connections, and access to resources.
- Identify potential candidates.
- Initiate a basic demographic and personal questionnaire to learn about the person's heritage, and past personal and professional experiences. If the candidate is married or partnered, conduct the same investigation of the candidate's partner.
- Administer a specialized questionnaire that focuses on the specific position for which the individual is being vetted.
- Conduct a background check that examines any illegal or criminal activity, or any interactions with the legal system.
- Examine all public records on the candidate.
- If the candidate is an elected official, scrutinize all previous votes on policies.
- Evaluate each public speech and critique all published reports and scholarly articles presented by the candidate.
- Conduct a personal financial background check to include all campaign contributions, income tax filings, employment of others, and investment strategies.

Political Campaigns

The activity of campaigning is a political strategy that can have multiple purposes. Some of the purposes of a campaign are to create name recognition and build a political base or constituency, influence others to vote for a specific candidate, frame an issue or problem, or educate constituents regarding policies. The political campaign strategy can include working on a political campaign or running a political campaign. **Table 10-22** presents guidelines for managing a political campaign. The three cardinal principles of campaigning are: know thyself, know thy voters, and know thy opponent.

Table 10-22 Campaign Guidelines

- Establish an exploration committee to evaluate potential for candidacy
  - o Examine the political environment
    - Analysis of constituency
    - Voter history
    - Opponent profiles
    - Concurrent political races
    - Media analysis
- Select a campaign manager
- Appoint a campaign committee
  - o Hire staff
  - o Develop campaign website
- Identify campaign strategy by writing a campaign plan
  - o Develop a platform
  - o Compose a brand and slogan
  - o Engage in opposition research
  - o Vet your opponent
  - o Public opinion polls, polling, and geomapping
  - o Examine campaign resources—time, money, people, and talent
  - o Secure campaign funding
  - o Fundraising
  - o Establish communication medium
  - o Identify "kitchen cabinet"
  - o Establish an advisory board
  - o Identify a spokesperson
  - o Plan to impact voter turnout, persuade voters
  - o Public appearances and speeches
  - o Grassroots efforts
  - o Secure endorsements and political party support
  - o Publicize campaign schedule and events
  - o Develop voter contact list
- Candidate development
  - o Listen and lead
  - o Meet opinion leaders
  - o Engage in grassroots activities
  - o Learn key media players
  - o Learn community organizations and special interest groups
  - o Polish personal communication skills and charisma

Debate

A debate is formal method of verbal argument. An argument for the purpose of a debate is a position with a justification or rationale that supports your assertion on the topic or issue. Most debates center on a controversial issue. The art of debate does not always rely solely on logic and reason, and can be used to educate the public, clarify issues, develop an agenda, assert a position on a topic, and persuade the audience in the direction of a specific policy or action. Therefore, debates also rely on appeal. The winning debater is the individual who presents the best argumentative framework regarding the issue being debated. There are various types of debates.

The four typical types of debates are parliamentary, Lincoln-Douglas, cross examination, and academic. A parliamentary debate requires no prior research on a policy issue. A parliamentary debate generally debates a resolution following accepted parliamentary procedures. Parliamentary debates rely heavily on logic, persuasiveness, and factual information. The Lincoln-Douglas debate is named after the original debate that occurred between Abe Lincoln and Stephen A. Douglas regarding slavery. A Lincoln-Douglas debate is generally a one-on-one debate between two individuals. A Lincoln-Douglas debate generally has two individuals who engage in a verbal argumentative dialogue regarding issues centered on moral issues, policy propositions, or values. The cross examination debate is also known as the policy debate, or the team debate. In a cross examination debate, one team presents an affirmative position regarding a policy issue and one team presents a negative position regarding the same policy issue. An academic debate is purely for academic enhancement. **Table 10-23** presents some general guidelines that may be used for a debate. **Table 10-24** presents a debate format.

Politics and Economics

Economics is the study of how individuals, groups, organizations, and societies allocate and use resources. In the policymaking process, policymakers make decisions regarding the costs and benefits of a policy solution or alternative. The two primary economic indicators in our country are the gross domestic product and the gross national product. The gross domestic product is the monetary total of all finished goods and services (public and private)

Table 10-23   Guideline for a Debate

- Debate preparation
  - o Prepare background information.
  - o Prepare a comprehensive bibliography and reference list to documents facts.
  - o Read a wide breadth of information on the topic.
  - o Prepare a debate strategy to frame the argument.
  - o Know your opponent's position and argument as well as you know your own position.
- In a team debate, each participant should speak.
- In a debate, each team or individual typically begins with a constructive speech which presents their basic position on the issue or policy agenda.
- Affirmative argument typically presented first
- Negative argument typically presents first rebuttal
- New constructive arguments are typically not introduced in the rebuttal period, unless it answers a direct question.
- Terms used should be well understood in terms of definition and intent.
- The individual who proposes an assertion in the debate is responsible for proving the assertion.
- Evidence and logic should support each assertion.
- Facts should be accurate.
- Restatement or a quotation of an opponent's argumentative statement must be accurate.
- Plans of action presented during a debate must be clearly outlined and explained.
- Debate rules should be established that define
  - o Time allotted for entire debate period
  - o Time allotted for the constructive introductory statements
  - o Time allotted to each speaker to present affirmative and negative statement
  - o Time allotted for each rebuttal
  - o Time allotted for closing statement
  - o Acceptable behavior during the debate
  - o Permissibility of visual aids during debate
  - o Determine if debate will have a rebuttal period and closing summary period or if the rebuttal period will serve as the closing summary.
- Avoid emotionally charged words.
- Exercise caution when asserting causal relationships.
- Avoid innuendo.
- Avoid rhetorical statements or the presentation of malevolent ideas.
- Do not commit *ad hominem*—attacking the presenter and not the argument.
- Do not assert your authority; argue with persuasion.
- Avoid pleading.
- Present a clear and consistent message.

Table 10-24   Debate Formats

General Format
- Constructive opening of affirmative
- Constructive opening of negative side
- First affirmative speech
- Question and answer period
- First negative speech
- Question and answer period
- Second affirmative speech
- Second negative speech
- Third affirmative speech

Lincoln-Douglas
- First affirmative constructive statement
- Cross examination of affirmative statements by negative side
- First negative constructive statement
- Cross examination of negative statements by affirmative side
- First affirmative rebuttal to negative side's argument
- Negative side rebuts the affirmative side's statements
- Second affirmative rebuttal (generally the final)

Lincoln-Douglas (Team Format)
- Each team member presents an affirmative or negative statement and responds once to the other team in the cross examination.
- First affirmative constructive statement
- Cross examination of affirmative statements by negative team
- First negative constructive statements
- Cross examination of negative teams by affirmative team
- Second affirmative constructive statement by another team member
- Cross examination of affirmative statement by another negative team member
- Second negative constructive by another team member
- Cross examination of negative statements by another affirmative team member
- First negative rebuttal
- First affirmative rebuttal
- Second negative rebuttal
- Second affirmative rebuttal (concludes debate)

produced within the nation in one year. The gross national product is the total market value of all goods and services produced in an economy during a period of time, which can be quarterly or yearly.

A frequent question for politicians regarding the policymaking process is whether to develop policy that redistributes existing resources or allocates new resources. All political and policy decisions have an economic impact if resources are necessary to implement the political or policy decision.

Politics and economics interact at two levels, microeconomic and macroeconomic. Microeconomics examines the allocation of resources at the individual decision-making level. In contrast, macroeconomics examines the allocation of resources at the aggregate national level. Whether politics and economics interact at the micro- or macroeconomic level, economic policy outcomes are generally judged according to the criteria of efficiency, equity, economic growth, and economic stability. Efficiency or allocative efficiency produces resources needed with the least possible cost. Equity refers to the fairness of the economic outcomes. Economic growth refers to an increase in the total output as the result of an economic decision. Economic stability is a state in which there are stable outputs with low inflation and maximum use of resources.

Political Analysis

Political analysis is the process of examining the political philosophy, and perspectives, structures, interactions, and networks that influence the policymaking process. The philosophical approaches that inform the political analysis process are empirical, normative, institutional, behavioral, and forces (internal and external). Empirical perspective uses observable data to analyze the political situation. The normative perspective focuses on what should be or ought to be the political activity in alignment with the espoused values. Institutional perspective analyzes the political activities in terms of the institutional culture and climate. Behavioral perspective attempts to explain, describe, and possibly predict the political behavior of individuals and groups. The forces perspective considers the internal and external forces that are exerted on an individual or group to influence their political activities (Heineman, 1996).

A political analysis examines the politics of the problem and the politics of the proposed policy. The steps of a political analysis are:

- Problem identification—This consists of determining the scope, duration, history, and sphere of impact of the problem.

- Analyzing proposed policy solutions—Each solution should be analyzed in respect to practicality, feasibility, potential outcomes, and resources needed.
- Background analysis of the problem—This analysis consists of the historical perspective of the problem, historical precedents, and past political actions with related policy problems and policy solutions.
- Identify the political structures supporting and opposing the policy solutions—This includes special interest groups, political parties, and policy precedents generated in the executive, legislative and judicial systems.
- Evaluate constituents—Examine who supports and opposes solutions, the presence of policy entrepreneurs, and the constituents' resource base.
- Conduct a values assessment.
- Evaluate the extent types of resources.
- Examine the constituents' power base.

Conflicts of Interest

A conflict of interest occurs when an individual has a conflict between personal or private interest and the responsibilities associated with their position of authority. Political activity can present many potential areas of conflict of interest. Chapter 11 provides information regarding conflicts of interest.

Lobbying and Government Employees

Employees of governmental agencies at the local, state, and national level may have employment-related restrictions in relation to lobbying and other types of political engagement. These requirements are typically a condition of employment. The employee does not forfeit their rights as a citizen but must be clear as to who they represent during their advocacy and lobbying efforts. An employee may act in self interest regarding an issue or problem to legislators but not as an agent of the employing organization. The rules and laws governing individual and organizational advocacy and lobbying activities differ. Therefore, it is vital that the respective individual is familiar with all applicable institutional, local, state, and federal laws governing individual and organizational level advocacy and lobbying activities.

Summary Points

- Political activity is a means to influence policymaking.
- Politics is defined as the process of influencing someone or something to ensure the allocation of resources as desired.
- Political astuteness refers to an understanding of different political agendas and power bases among various individuals, organizations, and institutions and the dynamic between them in relation to the proposed policy solution.
- Political power is the ability to exert control over the behavior of another.
- Political power can be considered potential or kinetic power.
- The monolithic paradigm model is an authoritarian framework with a fixed power structure.
- The pluralistic paradigm embraces power from a grassroots perspective, which originates from the people.
- The elements of power typically include instrumentalities (equipment, materials, funds), people, or information.
- Sources or types of political power can include: legitimate, reward, coercive, referent, expert, human resource, material, or charisma.
- Members of an iron triangle are congressional members, members of the executive branch of government, and special interest groups.
- Nurses' engagement in the policy process has been shaped by educational preparation, practice experience, professional engagement, and the maturity level of the nursing profession.
- The purpose of diagnosing organizational politics is to gain an understanding of the political structure and forces that effect policymaking changes within a defined organization.
- Organizational politics diagnosis identifies the influencing tactics.
- A political protocol consists of the written and unwritten rules that prescribe the appropriate manner of engaging with political and elected officials during formal functions and ceremonies.
- Liberals believe in the ownership of private property and use of natural resources for individual human gain.

- Socialism proposes shared property and wealth, and equal control and distribution of resources.
- The conservative perspective proposes that individuals with wealth and who are powerful in society have an obligation to provide resources and protect the less fortunate individuals in society.
- Five political system groups are: liberal democratic regimes, egalitarian-authoritarian, traditional-inegalitarian, populist, and authoritarian-inegalitarian.
- Political strategies are the methods and processes used to influence the desired policy goals.
- There are four primary types of conflict—intrapersonal, interpersonal, intergroup, and organizational.
- Lobbying is the process of approaching legislators or policymakers to present information to influence their decision making.
- Interest groups are groups of individuals or organizations that share political, social, or other common interests, that seek to influence the policymaking process.
- Seven functions of interest groups in our society are participation, representation, political education, motivation, mobilization, and monitoring of political behavior and policy
- The power of the media lies in the ability of editors, producers, anchors, reporters, and columnists to present policy problems or issues to the public within the public domain.
- Priming sets the stage for future messages regarding a policy problem or issue.
- Framing impacts the assimilation of information regarding a policy.
- Media analysis facilitates the assessment of the extent to which the information presented is biased or the manner in which the information is biased.
- Testimony is an oral presentation before a committee or official body either providing evidence, responding to questions, or presenting a position.
- Policy briefs provide a quick explanation of the policy issue or problem and the proposed policy, along with policy and political assessment.
- Policy speeches are conducted during political campaigns and during policy agenda setting and policymaking activities.

- A position paper typically describes the individual's or organization's position on an issue and a recommended solution with the supporting rationale for the position.
- A resolution is a formal motion, position, or solution proposed by an executive or governing body or organization.
- A resolution consists of four parts: heading, subject, preamble, and operative clause.
- Coalitions consolidate grassroots-level power and generate grassroots advocacy.
- Coalitions increase the political power structure by increasing the number of individuals supporting a specific policy.
- Political polls are surveys used to measure the potential of a specific candidate to win an election or to determine the level of support for a specific issue or policy.
- Public opinion is a good assessment of the national mood.
- Vetting is a process of conducting a comprehensive background examination and evaluation of an individual prior to appointing the person to a position or selecting the individual as a partner in a political campaign.
- A debate is a formal method of verbal argument.
- Policy, politics and economics are interrelated and inseparable.
- Economics is the study of how individuals, groups, organizations, and societies allocate and use resources.
- Political analysis is the process of examining the political philosophy, and perspectives, structures, interactions, and networks that influence the policymaking process.

References

Berkowitz, B., & Wolff, T. (2000). *The spirit of coalition*. Washington, DC: American Public Health Association.

Borkowski, N. (2005). *Organizational behavior in health care*. Sudbury, MA: Jones and Bartlett.

Britner, P., & Alpert, L. (2005). Writing *amicus curiae* and policy briefs: A pedagogical approach to teaching family law and policy. *Marriage & Family Review, 38*(2), 5–21.

Buppert, C. (2007). How to develop relationships with legislators. *The Journal of Nurse Practitioners, 3*(10), 682–683.

Buse, K., Mays, N., & Walt, G. (2005). *Making health policy*. Berkshire, England: Open University Press.

Cohen, S., Mason, D., Kovner, J., Pulcini, J., & Scholaski, J. (1996). Stages of nursing's political development: Where we've been and where we ought to go. *Nursing Outlook*, 44(6), 259–266.

Domke, D., Shah, D., & Wackman, D. (1998). Media priming effects: Accessibility, association, and activation. *International Journal of Public Opinion Research*, 10(1), 51–75.

Dye, T. (2010). *Understanding public policy* (13th ed.). Upper Saddle River, NJ: Prentice Hall.

Easton, D. (1965). *A systems analysis of political life*. New York, NY: Wiley.

Harrison, M., & Shirom, A. (1999). *Organizational diagnosis and assessment: Bridging theory and practice*. Thousand Oaks, CA: Sage Publications.

Heineman, R. (1996). *Political science: An introduction*. New York, NY: McGraw-Hill..

Jennings, C. (2002). The power of the policy brief. *Policy, Politics, & Nursing Practice*, 3(3), 261–263.

Kleinkauf, C. (1981). A guide to giving legislative testimony. *Social Work*, 26(4), 297–302.

Leavitt, J. (2009). Leaders in health policy: A critical role for nursing. *Nursing Outlook*, 57(2), 73–77.

Mason, D., Leavitt, J., & Chaffee, M. (2006). *Policy and politics in nursing and health care* (5th ed.). St. Louis, MO: Saunders.

Patterson, M. (2008). Nursing policy primer: Putting policy to work for your practice. *The Journal of Nurse Practitioners*, 4(10), 776–779.

Porche, D. (2003). *Public and community health nursing practice: A population-based approach*. Thousand Oaks, CA: Sage Publications

Prouty, J. (2000). *Agenda setting function of Maxwell McCombs & Donald Shaw*. Retrieved from http://oak.cats.ohiou.edu/~jp340497/agsapp.htm

Ridenour, J., & Harris, G. (2010). Shaping public policy: The nurse regulator's role. *Journal of Nursing Regulation*, 1(1), 26–29.

Scholzman, K., Burns, N., & Verba, S. (1994). Gender and the pathways to participation: The roles of resources. *Journal of Politics*, 65(4), 963-990.

Smith, K., & Larimer, C. (2009). *The public policy theory primer*. Boulder, CO: Westview Press.

Thomas, K., & Kilmann, R. (2002). *Thomas-Kilmann conflict mode instrument*. Palo Alto, CA: CPP.

Verba, S., Scholzman, K., & Brady, H. (1995). *Voice and equality: Civic voluntarism in American politics*. Cambridge, MA: Harvard University Press.

Policy, Law, and Politics: Ethical Perspective

The public expects accountability in all aspects of governmental relations. Elected officials and their representatives and delegates are expected to avoid conflicts of interest in the policymaking process. Ethical behavior and political activity are two behaviors that can co-exist and are not mutually exclusive concepts. The public expects policymakers, constituents, and policy implementers to behave in an ethical manner. In addition, expectations of accountability have been strengthened within the business community, requiring institutional and organizational policies to be formulated and implemented in an ethical manner. This chapter presents an overview of ethics to facilitate ethical policymaking and political activity.

Ethics Defined

Ethics is defined as the study of the nature and justification of principles that guide individuals to act in a moral manner that is consistent with society's customs, values, beliefs, and norms. Ethics is also described as the study of the manner in which individuals behave in a situation or as the basis for determining correct action. The field of ethics continues to evolve as societal needs change, technological advancements occur, and policies evolve (Porche, 2003).

Professional ethics "seek out the values and standards that have been developed by practitioners and leaders of a given profession over a long period of time and ... identify those values that seem most salient and inherent" to the professional discipline (Callahan & Jennings, 2002, p. 172). Applied ethics adopts a point of view that promotes practical application in real-world ethical issues. Applied ethics focuses more on professional behavior and conduct in specific situations based on the values of a profession (Callahan & Jennings, 2002). Advocacy ethics focuses equality and social justice. There are basic theoretical frameworks that guide ethical decision-making (Beauchamp & Childress, 2008). Other essential ethics terms are presented in **Table 11-1**.

Table 11-1   Ethical Terminology

Ethics	Process of determining right and wrong conduct
Morals	Qualities that are considered by society to be associated with being intrinsically good
Unethical	An action or conduct that violates ethical principles, accepted values, or morals
Ethical gray area	An ethical situation or problem that does not neatly fit into any one specific categorization
Cognitive dissonance	A cognitive process in which there is a discrepancy between what a person believes, knows, and values, and what is perceived to be true and real. The individual attempts to bring behavior in alignment to avoid the discomfort created by the dissonance.
Altruism	The regard for others
Beneficence	The principle that one should assist others; to do good
Duty	An action or act that must occur because of a moral or legal obligation
Egoism	Self promotion is the sole objective
Equality	Equal distribution
Liberty	Freedom of human action; grounded in principle of autonomy
Veracity	Principle of truth telling
Vices	Negative ethical or character traits
Virtues	Positive ethical or character traits

Ethical Theories and Paradigms

Ethical theories are the frameworks that provide the context in which an individual engages in ethical decision making. Ethical theories serve as guidelines to assist with the analysis of ethical dilemmas, and guide an individual in determining ethical actions. Two classical ethical theories are deontology and utilitarianism.

Deontology

Deontology is a theoretical framework based on a sense of moral obligation or duty. Deontology states that an action's moral rightness or wrongness depends on the action itself and the motivation behind the action (Beauchamp & Childress, 2008). Deontology acknowledges the moral obligation that individuals feel toward certain actions. Moral obligation refers to an individual feeling a sense of duty that requires them to act in a particular manner in response to their values, beliefs, and perspective of societal norms.

Utilitarianism

Teleology is an ethical theory that determines rightness or wrongness based solely on the expected outcomes or consequences of an action. Utilitarianism is a theoretical framework of teleology theory. The utilitarian framework proposes that the most ethical action is that which results in the greatest good for the largest number of individuals (Beauchamp & Childress, 2008). Utilitarianism does not specifically focus on the action but on the ultimate number of individuals impacted by the action.

Ethical Principles

Ethical principles evolve from an individual's guiding ethical theoretical perspective, personal paradigm regarding moral conduct, and societal expectations. Ethical theories in addition to the moral tone of society assist in the formulation of ethical principles that guide an individual's ethical behavior. In addition, ethical principles are the foundation of professional codes of ethics. Ethical principles guide an individual in the critical analysis and reasoning of an ethical dilemma. The most common principles encountered in ethics are beneficence, nonmaleficence, justice, and autonomy (Beauchamp & Childress, 2008).

Beneficence consists of norms providing the greatest benefit to an individual, group, or community. Beneficence consists of weighing the benefits of an action against the risks or costs to the individual, group, or community involved (Beauchamp & Childress, 2008).

Nonmaleficence is the ethical principle of "doing no harm." With nonmaleficence, the policymaker focuses on not causing harm to individuals, groups, or communities. (Beauchamp & Childress, 2008).

Justice is the ethical principle of ensuring the fair and equitable distribution of benefits, risks, and cost. Justice is known as the ethical principle of fairness (Beauchamp & Childress, 2008).

Autonomy is the ethical principle known as "respect for persons." Autonomy provides individuals with the right to make their own autonomous decisions. This is also referred to as the right to self-determination. This principle provides individuals with the right to make free, uncoerced, and informed decisions. Autonomy is the ethical principle that provides the framework of full disclosure and informed consent (Beauchamp & Childress, 2008).

In addition to the ethical principles of beneficence, nonmaleficence, justice, and autonomy, fidelity and veracity are two other principles essential in ethical decision-making processes. Fidelity is known as promise keeping. Fidelity ensures that the policymaker delivers what was promised in the form of policy. Veracity is known as truth telling. Veracity consists of being honest in delivering information to a policymakers constituency. Fidelity and veracity are essential for a policymaker to develop a trusting relationship with constituents.

Values Clarification

Values are beliefs that an individual or social group has regarding what is relevant and important to their belief system. Values generally have an emotional attachment. Values are continually formed throughout life as an individual develops, and as the contextual and social situation of the individual changes. Some values are permanent and some values transform as an individual grows and develops. Value formation originates within the individual's family unit and continues to evolve with socialization into different professional and societal groups. Values that typically do not change, and form the basis for other values and philosophical perspectives are considered core values. An individual's values comprise the belief system or framework that structures the manner in which an individual views the world. In other words, this value system serves as the framework that creates an individual's paradigm regarding policy and politics (Coletta, 1978).

Values form the foundation for ethical decisions. To engage in moral thoughts and actions, an individual needs to have a framework of values that comprise their professional and personal life. The value clarification process promotes clarity regarding an individual's personal and professional values that form the foundation for their thoughts and actions in relation to policy and politics.

The value clarification process promotes self-reflection to identify an individual's values and value system. During this process of self-reflection, the policymaker has the ability to analyze and prioritize the values that compose their value system through a process of refinement. Raths et al. (1966) defined a seminal process of values clarification. The process consists of choosing, prizing, and acting. In accordance with this process, a value is that which meets more than two criteria resulting from these three processes (see **Figure 11-1**).

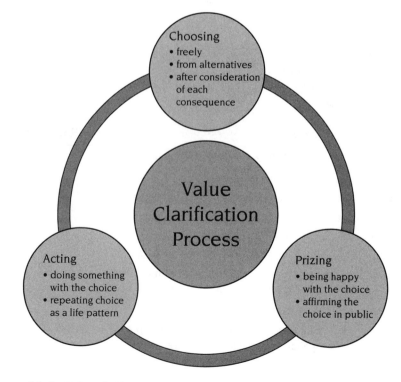

Figure 11-1 Value clarification process

Choosing consists of three criteria. These criteria are: choosing freely, choosing from alternatives (thoughts and actions), and choosing after thoughtful consideration of the consequences of each alternative. The next process, prizing, consists of two criteria. These two criteria are cherishing and being happy with the choice, and willingness to affirm the choice within a public arena. Lastly, the acting process is defined by doing something with the choice, and repeatedly acting in the same manner as a life pattern. Collectively, these three processes define the value clarification process that identifies an individual's values which comprise their personal and professional policymaking paradigm. **Table 11-2** provides a value clarification exercise to assist an individual with determining the values that comprise their value system. This process of self-reflection increases an individual's personal understanding and self-awareness.

Table 11-2   Values Clarification Exercise

The following is a list of personal and professional values. Carefully consider each value. Rate each value using the following scale:

1 = Not at all important to me
2 = Not very important to me
3 = Moderately important to me
4 = Very important to me
5 = Essential to me

Value	Meaning	Rating (1 to 5)
Achievement	Accomplishment of a desired goal	
Aesthetics	Appreciation for beauty	
Altruism	A genuine regard and devotion to the interest of others	
Autonomy	Freedom of self-determination	
Diversity	Appreciation for differences or variation	
Emotional well-being	Freedom from anxiety; piece of mind; inner feelings of pleasure	
Excellence	Highest quality	
Family	Maintain strong sense of relationship to genetic relatives or group of choice	

(continues)

Table 11-2   Values Clarification Exercise (*continued*)

Value	Meaning	Rating (1 to 5)
Health	Freedom from disease or pain; general condition of well-being	
Honesty	Being truthful; straightforwardness of conduct	
Integrity	Quality of having high moral principles, being reliable and trustworthy	
Justice	Quality of being impartial, just and fair	
Knowledge	Attainment of information or truth, power of knowing	
Love	Affection or admiration for another	
Loyalty	Maintaining an allegiance to a person, institution, political body, or another entity	
Morality	Belief in and maintenance of ethical standards	
Pleasure	An agreeable emotion of satisfaction or gratification	
Power	Ability to influence others or exert control	
Professionalism	Adherence to a set of values comprising statutory professional obligations, formally agreed codes of conduct, and the informal expectations aligned with the respective discipline	
Recognition	Providing attention as a means to convey significance and importance	
Respect	Positive feeling of esteem or admiration for another person or entity; deference toward another person or entity	
Security	A feeling of safety or comfort	
Skill	Ability to execute a specific technical expertise	
Spirituality	Belief in or feeling of connection with a higher being	
Wealth	An abundance of material possessions or resources	
Wisdom	Insight, good sense, good judgment, intuitive knowledge	

Ethical Decision-making Process

An ethical dilemma arises when there is a conflict in the principles, duties, rights, beliefs, or values of one individual, group, population, or community with another or with societal expectations (Beauchamp & Childress, 2008). A reflective process that generates solutions or alternatives to the ethical dilemma is known as the ethical decision-making process.

Ethical decision-making processes facilitate the selection of an ethical resolution by outlining the steps that promote an understanding of the ethical dilemma and the preferred resolution. Ethical theoretical perspective and ethical principles are used in the ethical decision-making process to analyze the ethical dilemma. There are several decision-making processes that can be used to assist with ensuring that an individual selects the most ethical behavior within the given contextual situation. The two processes presented next are similar, but differ in the method by which the final ethical decision is rendered.

Porche (2003) proposed the following steps as a reflective process to reason through an ethical dilemma:

1. Define the ethical dilemma.
2. Outline the conflicting ethical issues and principles resulting from both sides of the ethical dilemma.
3. Identify the constituency impacted at all policy levels and on both sides of the dilemma.
4. Collect data relevant to both sides of the ethical dilemma.
5. List alternative policy options to resolve the ethical dilemma.
6. Describe the consequences for each policy option listed.
7. Analyze each policy option in relation to the preferred ethical theoretical paradigm, and ethical principles or codes of ethics.
8. Determine which policy option would be the best and most ethical resolution.
9. Draft policy that represents the ethical resolution selected.
10. Ensure that the policy is implemented with the ethical intent and context that provided the framework to develop the policy.
11. Evaluate the implementation and consequences of the ethical resolution. Consider the impact of the ethical resolution on each constituency.

An ethical decision-making process has been proposed by the Josephson Institute of Ethics. This decision-making process consists of five principled reasoning steps: These five steps are:

1. Clarification
   a. Determine what must be decided.
   b. Formulate a full range of alternative decision.
   c. Eliminate any alternative decisions that have any unethical actions.
   d. Prioritize the decisions hierarchically in relation to ethical principles.
2. Evaluate—Consider all decisions in terms of practicality, ethics, benefits, burdens, and risk to all individuals involved.
3. Decide
   a. Make the best decision based on personal conscience and appropriateness of action.
   b. Consider the following: Are you treating others as you would want to be treated? Would you be comfortable if your reasoning and decision were to be made public? Would you be comfortable if your children were observing your behavior?
4. Implement
   a. Develop a plan to implement the decisions.
   b. Maximize benefits while reducing cost and risks.
5. Modify and Monitor
   a. Evaluate and adjust the plan to new information.
   b. Monitor the effects of the decisions.
   c. Revise plan of action based on new information (Josephson Institute of Ethics, 1999).

Codes of Ethics

Codes of ethics are derived from normative ethics. Ethical codes are used to transmit moral guidelines of discipline or professional group. These ethical codes represent the values inherent in a profession or professional group (Beauchamp & Childress, 2008).

Ethical Engagement in Political Process

Engagement in the political process is expected to be ethical. Political plans should create an ethical infrastructure within the plan. This ethical infrastructure should ensure that there is a system of checks and balances that occur with the execution of each political strategy. This promotes integrity, transparency, and accountability within the political process of policymaking. This means that the ethical decision-making process should be executed when discerning among political strategies selected. However, prior to the working of the political action plan, the individuals involved in the decision making and implementation of political strategies must identify and clearly understand their values and guiding ethical principles.

Government Employees and Ethics

Government employees and elected officials are expected to engage in ethical behavior and conduct the affairs of their offices in an ethical manner. Government employees, regardless of the branch of government (executive, legislative or judicial) should hold their positions of public trust in high regard. The American people have a right to expect that all government employees will be loyal to the Constitution (or state constitutions or city charters), laws, regulations, ethical principles and codes of ethics. **Tables 11-3** and **11-4** provide codes of ethical conduct for lobbying and government service.

Table 11-3   Code of Lobbying Ethics

Lobbyists are expected to demonstrate the highest ethical conduct during lobbying efforts. The American League of Lobbyists provides the following code of ethics for independent lobbyists. This code of ethics can provide a framework for all individuals engaged in lobbying activities. The American League of Lobbyist Code of Ethics is summarized below:

- Honesty and integrity
  - ○ Truthful in communicating with public officials.
  - ○ Provide accurate and factual information.
  - ○ Ensure that new accurate and updated information is provided if any information that was provided becomes inaccurate.
- Compliance with applicable laws, regulations, and rules
  - ○ Be familiar with laws, regulations, and rules.
  - ○ Do not cause self or public officer to violate any law, regulation, or rule.
- Professionalism
  - ○ Act in a fair and professional manner.
  - ○ Acquire knowledge of legislative and governmental processes.

(continues)

Table 11-3   Code of Lobbying Ethics (*continued*)

- ○ Represent clients in a competent and professional manner.
- ○ Engage in continuing education to understand legislative and governmental processes.
- ○ Treat others with respect and civility.
- Conflicts of interest
  - ○ Do not engage in representation that creates conflicts of interest without all parties involved having full disclosure through an informed consent process.
  - ○ Avoid advocating a position while representing another client on the same issue with a conflicting position.
  - ○ Obtain consent from a client if representation of one client on an issue may have a significant adverse impact on another client's interest.
  - ○ Disclose all potential conflicts to current and prospective clients and disclose methods to resolve conflicts of interest with all parties.
  - ○ Inform all clients when receiving a direct or indirect referral or consulting fee from the lobbyist in connection with the client's work.
- Due diligence and best efforts
  - ○ Devote adequate time, attention, and resources to lobbying efforts.
  - ○ Exercise loyalty.
  - ○ Keep client informed regarding your work activities on their behalf.
- Compensation and engagement terms
  - ○ Retain clients using a written agreement specifying the terms and conditions of the agreement.
  - ○ Cite basis for compensation, fees, and other expenditures in which compensation is required.
- Confidentiality
  - ○ Do not disclose confidential and privileged information without the client's expressed consent.
  - ○ Do not use confidential information against the interest of any other parties.
- Public education
  - ○ Ensure the public understands and appreciates the nature, legitimacy, and necessity of lobbying.
- Duty to governmental institutions
  - ○ Respect all governmental institutions.
  - ○ Do not undermine public confidence and trust in the democratic governmental process.
  - ○ Do not act in any manner that demonstrates disrespect for governmental institutions.

Source: American League of Lobbyists. (2010). *Code of ethics.* Retrieved from http://www.alldc.org/ethicscode.cfm

Table 11-4   United States Government Service Code of Ethics

Any person in government service should:

I.   Put loyalty to the highest moral principles above loyalty to persons, party, or government department.

II.   Uphold the Constitution, laws, and legal regulations of the United States and of all governments therein and never be a party to their evasion.

III.   Give a full day's labor for a full day's pay; giving to the performance of his duties his earnest effort and best thought.

IV.   Seek to find and employ more efficient and economical ways of getting tasks accomplished.

V.   Never discriminate unfairly by the dispensing of special favors or privileges to anyone, whether for remuneration or not; and never accept, for himself or his family, favors or benefits under circumstances which might be construed by reasonable persons as influencing the performance of his governmental duties.

VI.   Make no private promises of any kind binding upon the duties of office, since the government employee has no private word which can be binding on public duty.

VII.   Engage in no business with the government, either directly or indirectly, which is inconsistent with the conscientious performance of his governmental duties.

VIII. Never use any information coming to him confidentially in the performance of governmental duties as a means for making private profit.

IX.   Expose corruption wherever discovered.

X.   Uphold these principles, ever conscious that public office is a public trust.

Source: H.R. Doc. No. 64-103 (1958).

In 1989, President George H. W. Bush issued Executive Order 12674 (which was then modified in 1990 by Executive Order 12731), that outlined general principles broadly defining the obligation of public service. Two core concepts provided the basis for these principles:

- Employees shall not use their public office for private gain.
- Employees shall act impartially and not give preferential treatment to any private organization or individual.

In addition, these executive orders strongly encouraged that employees avoid any action that would create the appearance of violating the law or ethical standards. President Bush was striving to generate public confidence and trust in the integrity of government operations and programs. Other recommended cautions to not misuse a position in the executive branch of government consisted of:

- Employees are not to use their position, title, or any authority associated with their office to coerce or induce a benefit for self, family, or friends.
- Employees are not to use or allow the improper use of nonpublic information to advance the private interest of themselves or their acquaintances.
- Use government property only for authorized purposes.
- Employees may not misuse official paid time.

A great concern in relation to the ethical behavior of governmental employees involves financial conflicts of interest. The following strategies are suggested to avoid potential financial conflicts of interest:

- Recusals—Do not participate in any matter that poses a conflict of interest.
- Waivers—Secure a waiver from the appropriate authorized official.
- Divestiture—Sell or separate legally from any property or financial interest that may appear to be a financial conflict of interest. A "certificate of divestiture" may be required from the appropriate authorized official.
- Trusts—Develop trusts in accordance with the Internal Revenue Code.

Governmental employees are encouraged build public trust through the creation of transparent activities. Transparency is a key leadership strategy for building trust within organizations and among constituents. The following are recommendations to facilitate the development of transparency and to ultimately build trust:

- Communicate in a meaningful, purposive, unpretentious, and clear manner presenting factual information with full disclosure.
- Provide access to information within a public arena. This information can be limited to the internal citizens of an organization.
- Publicize areas of responsibility and accountability among the administrative team.
- Reveal information regarding yourself that is pertinent to your position and activities.

- Disclose any apparent, potential, or actual conflicts of interest.
- Limit interlinking of personal and professional relationships, if they are present, ensure that the exact nature of the relationship is known.
- Encourage open meetings, publicize closed "executive" sessions prior to the meetings.
- Publicize meeting agendas.
- Have an open door policy.
- Have open meetings with no agenda and encourage open questions and dialogue.
- Publicize strategic vision, mission, and strategic plans. Consider posting action plans of the strategic plan.
- Provide access to outcome and other evaluation data.
- Ensure that the fiscal management has an open process that provides individuals with access to the organization's financial data.

Conflict of Interest

Transparency is one means to avoid conflicts of interest. A conflict of interest occurs when an individual has a conflict between personal or private interest and the responsibilities associated with their position of authority. Conflicts of interest do not only pertain to financial benefits. Conflict of interest does not always have to be actual with tangible outcomes but conflict of interest can exist even if others perceive that there is the appearance of a conflict of interest. There are several types of conflicts of interest: objective, subjective, potential, actual, or apparent. An objective conflict of interest involves a financial relationship. A subjective conflict of interest is based on emotional ties or a relationship. A potential conflict of interest occurs when an individual has an interest that may influence their judgment and decisions in the future. An actual conflict of interest occurs when an individual has an interest that impacts their judgment and they engaged in an activity that is directly related to the area of the conflict. An apparent conflict of interest occurs when there is no actual conflict of interest but other persons looking at the situation perceive that there is an actual conflict of interest (Velasquez, 2006). An individual's employment position, profession, and personal obligations and responsibilities influence conflicts of interest.

Regardless of the type of conflict, engagement in a conflict of interest activity is considered unethical behavior. The best strategy regarding conflicts of interest is to prevent or avoid an actual or perceived conflict of interest. The following measures are recommended to avoid conflict of interest:

- Maintain role clarity.
- Act in accordance with rules and regulations.
- Follow the letter and intent or spirit of the policy.
- Recognize potential conflicts of interest early.
- Identify primary and secondary constituents of a potential conflict of interest.
- Examine and reflect on any potential conflict of interest.
- Review policies governing potential conflicts of interest.
- Discuss potential conflicts of interest with individuals whose span of authority encompasses the area of potential conflict.
- Secure an opinion regarding the potential conflict of interest prior to engaging in an activity that may be determined a conflict of interest.

Summary Points

- The public expects accountability in all aspects of governmental relations.
- Ethics is defined as the study of the nature and justification of principles that guide individuals to act in a moral manner that is consistent with society's customs, values, beliefs, and norms.
- Professional ethics "seek out the values and standards that have been developed by practitioners and leaders of a given profession over a long period of time and … identify those values that seem most salient and inherent" to the professional discipline.
- Applied ethics adopts a point of view that promotes practical application in real-world ethical issues.
- Deontology states that an action's moral rightness or wrongness depends on the action itself and the motivation behind the action.
- The utilitarian framework proposes that the most ethical action is that which results in the greatest good for the largest number of individuals,
- The most common principles encountered in ethics are beneficence, nonmaleficence, justice, and autonomy.
- Beneficence consists of weighing the benefits of an action against the risks or costs to the individual, group, or community involved.

- Nonmaleficence is the ethical principle of "doing no harm."
- Justice is the principle of being fair and equitable.
- The principle of autonomy provides individuals with the right to make free, uncoerced, and informed decisions.
- The value clarification process promotes clarity regarding an individual's personal and professional values that form the foundation for their thoughts and actions in relation to policy and politics.
- The value clarification process promotes self-reflection to identify an individual's values and value system.
- Ethical decision-making processes facilitate the selection of an ethical resolution by outlining the steps that promote an understanding of the ethical dilemma and the preferred resolution.
- Transparency is a strategy to avoid conflicts of interest and promote trust.

References

American League of Lobbyists. (2010). *Code of ethics*. Retrieved from http://www.alldc.org/ethicscode.cfm

Beauchamp, T., & Childress, J. (2008). *Principles of biomedical ethics* (6th ed.). New York, NY: Oxford University Press.

Callahan, D., & Jennings, B. (2002). Ethics and public health: Forging a strong relationship. *American Journal of Public Health*, 92(2), 169–176.

Coletta, S. (1978). Value clarification in nursing: Why? *American Journal of Nursing*, 78(12), 2057.

Josephson Institute of Ethics. (1999). *Five steps of principled reasoning*. Retrieved from http://www.cs.bgsu.edu/maner/heuristics/1999JosephsonInstitute.htm

H.R. Doc. No. 64-103 (1958).

Porche, D. (2003). *Public and community health nursing practice: A population-based approach*. Thousand Oaks, CA: Sage Publications.

Raths, L., Harmin, M., & Simon, S. (1966). *Values and teaching*. Columbus, OH: Charles E. Merill.

Velasquez, M. (2006). *Business ethics: Concepts and cases* (6th ed.). Upper Saddle River, NJ: Prentice Hall.

Policy Institutes

Policy institutes are organizations that engage in a variety of policy activities that impact the policymaking process, policy analysis, policy research, or policy evaluation. Policy institutes are generally nonprofit and nonpartisan. Some policy institute organizations have a membership base. A policy institute with a membership base may also serve as a special interest group. Policy institutes may have resources (human, physical, or fiscal) that can be mobilized to engage in political activities to influence the policymaking process. Each policy institute has its own policy agenda. Policy institutes influence policy through conducting policy analysis and evaluating existing policies. These policy institutes typically have a repertoire of information regarding the issues on their policy agenda. Therefore, policy institutes serve a critical role as an information source for policy analysis and policy evaluation. In addition, the policy institute can be mobilized to politically influence the policymaking process. Familiarity with policy institutes is encouraged. The following is a partial list of well-known policy institutes. See Appendix C for more information.

American Association of Retired Persons (AARP) Public Policy Institute

The American Association of Retired Persons (AARP) Public Policy Institute is a component of the national organization American Association of Retired Persons. AARP is a nonprofit, nonpartisan membership-based organization that provides assistance to persons 50 years of age and older to improve their quality of life. Topics of interest for the AARP Public Policy Institute include consumer protection (financial services, financial literacy, fraud and deception, energy and public utilities, telecommunications, advance planning, and legal rights), economic security (social security, pensions and retirement savings, income and assets, tax and budget, work and retirement, low-income programs), health care (Medicare, Medicaid, health costs, health coverage and insurance, health quality, patient safety, access to care, health behaviors, prescription drugs, healthcare workforce, and nursing), livable communities (housing and transportation), and long-term care issues (assisted living, caregiving, home health, community-based care, long-term care insurance, nursing homes). AARP Public Policy Institute activities include program development, policy research, educational conferences, production of surveys, development of educational media and information to inform the public, and generation of policy reports.

American Enterprise Institute for Public Policy Research

The American Enterprise Institute for Public Policy Research is a private, nonpartisan, not-for-profit organization dedicated to research and education on government, politics, economics, and social welfare issues. This institute engages in policy research, open debate, and reasoned argument regarding the institute's primary areas of interest. Research is conducted in six primary areas: economic policy studies, foreign and defense policy studies, health policy studies, legal and constitutional studies, political and public opinion studies, and social and cultural studies. This institute engages in its work through specialized programs such as the Brandy Program on Culture and Freedom, Center for Regulatory and Market Studies, and the National Research Initiative. A host of experts, scholars, officers, and fellows conduct the activities of this institute.

Aspen Institute

The Aspen Institute's mission is to foster values-based leadership and to promote a neutral and balanced venue for discussion and acting on critical issues. Activities of the Aspen Institute include but are not limited to conducting seminars; sponsoring young leader fellowships; engaging nonpartisan forums for policy analysis; consensus building and problem solving in relation to policy issues; and sponsoring public conferences to share ideas and engage in debate. The Aspen Institute strives to create an enlightened population regarding critical issues.

Brookings Institution

The Brookings Institution is a nonprofit public policy organization. The mission of the Brookings Institution is to conduct high-quality and independent research to provide innovative, practical recommendations that advance the Brookings Institution's goals. The goals are: to strengthen the American democracy; foster economic and social welfare; promote security and opportunity for all Americans; and secure an open, safe, prosperous and cooperative international system. Members of the Brookings Institution write books, papers, articles and opinion pieces, and testify before congressional committees on various issues.

Cato Institute

The Cato Institute is a nonprofit public policy research foundation. The Cato Institute focuses on increasing the understanding of public policies with the premise of limited government, free markets, individual liberty, and peace. The Institute originates, advocates, promotes, and disseminates policy proposals for a free, open, and civil society in the United States and the world. The work of the Cato Institute is achieved through several centers: constitutional studies, educational freedom, global liberty and prosperity, representative government, trade policy studies, federal government downsizing, and social security choice.

Center for Responsive Politics

The Center for Responsive Politics conducts research on congressional and political trends. The center focuses on the specific areas of campaign finance, government ethics, political foundations, public policy, the media and Congress, and the inner workings of Congress.

Claremont Institute for Economic Policy Studies

The Claremont Institute for Economic Policy Studies conducts policy research and analysis on domestic and international economic policy issues. This institute exists in partnership with Claremont McKenna College. Major research focus areas include economic growth, inflation, migration, currency, and financial crisis.

The Commonwealth Fund

The Commonwealth Fund is a private foundation. The specific aims of the Commonwealth Fund are to promote a high-performing healthcare system to achieve the primary outcomes of better access, improved quality, and greater efficiency. The Commonwealth Fund focuses on the most vulnerable members of society such as low-income, uninsured, and minority Americans, young children, and elderly adults. The Commonwealth Fund's work includes a commission on high-performance health systems, the future of health insurance, state innovations, Medicare's future, healthcare quality improvement and efficiency, patient-centered primary care initiative, healthcare disparities, child development and preventive care, quality of care for frail elders, and the international program in health policy and practice. The Commonwealth Fund engages in policy research, produces reports, and funds grants.

Economic Policy Institute

The Economic Policy Institute is a nonprofit think tank organization that promotes discussion about economic policy. This organization focuses on the economic issues that impact both low- and middle-income workers. The Economic Policy Institute engages in policy research, policy analysis, community outreach and education. The economic issues of focus include but are not limited to: wages, incomes, prices, health care, education, retirement security, state-level economic development, trade and global finance, comparative international economic performance, manufacturing, global competitiveness, and energy development. The products of the Economic Policy Institute consist of books, studies, issue briefs, education materials, conferences and seminars, technical support, local activism, and testimony.

The Educational Policy Institute

The Educational Policy Institute's mission is to expand educational opportunities for low-income and historically under-represented students. The Educational Policy Institute engages in policy research and analysis. A goal of the Educational Policy Institute is to generate policy research and analysis that increases the number of students prepared for, enrolled in, and completing postsecondary educational programs. The competencies of this Institute are program evaluation, policy analysis, professional development, research design and management, and data services. Research areas of the Institute are early childhood, students with disabilities, teacher preparation and development, early intervention and outreach, student graduation and retention, student aid and access, retention and success, quality measurement in higher education, and university rankings.

Fairness and Accuracy in Reporting

Fairness and Accuracy in Reporting is a liberal media organization. This organization attempts to review the accuracy of media reports. The desire is to expose conservative bias in the media. Fairness and Accuracy in Reporting produces a magazine, newsletter, and a nationally syndicated weekly radio program.

Hudson Institute

The Hudson Institute is a nonpartisan policy research organization that conducts innovative research and policy analysis. The focus of the Hudson

Institute includes global security, prosperity, and freedom. The activities of the Hudson Institute are producing policy publications, sponsoring conferences, and publishing policy recommendations. The current research agenda for the Hudson Institute includes global affairs; science, environment, and technology; law, culture, and society; international governance; and economics and energy policy.

Institute for Higher Education Policy (IHEP)

The Institute for Higher Education Policy (IHEP) is an independent, nonprofit organization focused on access and success in postsecondary education around the world. IHEP engages in research and innovative program development as a means to inform policymakers' decision making processes and shape public policy. IHEP supports economic and social development through policy initiatives in postsecondary education. The vision of IHEP is a world in which all people achieve their full potential by participating and succeeding in postsecondary education. The five focus areas of IHEP are access and success, accountability, diversity, finance, and global impact. IHEP serves as a nonpartisan global research and policy center for government agencies, higher education organizations, philanthropic foundations, and other organizations with an interest in postsecondary education access and success. The activities of IHEP include policy research, policy analysis, composing professional reports and briefings, and program evaluation.

Institute for Philosophy and Public Policy

The Institute for Philosophy and Public Policy investigates the conceptual and ethical aspects of public policy formulation and debate. The institute explores the philosophical issues that influence constituents and policymakers.

Justice Policy Institute

The Justice Policy Institute promotes alternatives to incarceration of the prison population. The mission of the Justice Policy Institute is to promote effective solutions to societal problems and to end society's reliance on incarceration of prisoners. The Justice Policy Institute engages in: developing policy briefs, policy reports, and research projects; strategic communications and media advocacy; providing technical assistance and consultation; providing training on research and communications; and rapid response initiatives relating to emerging issues of incarceration.

Kaiser Family Foundation

The Kaiser Family Foundation is a nonprofit, private foundation. This foundation focuses on major healthcare issues in the United States and the country's role in impacting global health. The Kaiser Family Foundation serves as an information source that provides facts and information to inform policy analysis and policy research. This foundation serves as the "go to" organization for policy information. The foundation works in three primary areas: health policy; media and public education; and health and development in South Africa.

Kettering Foundation

The Kettering Foundation is a nonprofit research organization. The Kettering Foundation conducts research in the areas of community, governing, politics, and education. A special focus area of the Kettering Foundation is deliberative democracy.

National Institute for Public Policy

The National Institute for Public Policy is a nonprofit public education organization. This institute's policy agenda focuses on US foreign defense policies and international policy issues. Areas of specific focus for this institute are: international security issues; proliferation of missiles and weapons of mass destruction; effectiveness of post-Cold War deterrence theory; North Atlantic Treaty Organization (NATO); US–Russian political and military relations; evolution of arms control regimes; future of US strategic forces and role of nuclear weapons; roles and missions of the US intelligence community; role of air power; role of ballistic missile defense; and space power and policy studies.

Rand Corporation

The Rand Corporation is a nonprofit, independent, institution focused on improving policy and policy decision making through the conducting of policy research and policy analysis. The following issues are of primary importance to the Rand Corporation: health, education, national security, international affairs, law and business, and the environment. The core research areas of the Rand Corporation are the arts, child policy, civil justice, education, energy and environment, health and health care, international affairs, national security, population and aging, public safety, science and technology, substance abuse, terrorism and homeland security, transportation and infrastructure, and the workforce and workplace.

Robert Wood Johnson Foundation

The Robert Wood Johnson Foundation strives to improve the health and health care of all Americans. The targeted portfolio focuses on these program areas: building human capital, childhood obesity, available and equitable health coverage, support for pioneering innovations, public health services, and vulnerable populations.

The Rockefeller Foundation

The Rockefeller Foundation provides funding to support the goal of improving the well-being of humanity through smart globalization. The Rockefeller Foundation seeks to: nurture innovation; pioneer new fields; expand access to and improve distribution of resources; empower beneficiaries; and to generate a sustainable impact on individuals, institutions, and communities. The five policy issue areas for the Rockefeller Foundation include basic survival safeguards, global health, climate and environment, urbanization, and social and economic security. This foundation focuses its resources and provides funding for these five related issues that are linked and interlinked. Initiatives to impact these five policy areas include developing climate change resilience; strengthening food security; protecting American workers' economic security; promoting equitable sustainable transportation; linking global disease surveillance networks; transforming health systems; harnessing the power of impact investing; advancing innovation processes to solve social problems, the New York City fund, and assisting in the rebuilding of New Orleans post-Katrina.

Schneider Institutes for Health Policy

The Schneider Institutes for Health Policy is a group of policy research institutes within Brandeis University's Heller School of Social Policy and Management. The mission of the Schneider Institutes for Health Policy is to conduct health services research and engage in policy efforts focusing on healthcare financing and service delivery; the relationship between health services, behavior and socio-economic characteristics; and the connection between health status and individual and societal well-being. The research focuses on three areas: acute and chronic health care, behavioral health, and international health. The institute has core competency and experts in six areas: financing, organizing, cost and value, quality, high risk and costly populations, and technology. The three populations of significance to this Institute are the elderly, individuals with chronic illness, and individuals with substance abuse and mental health issues.

Urban Institute

The Urban Institute is a result of a blue ribbon commission of civic leaders that encouraged the development of an independent, nonpartisan organization. This occurred at the recommendation of President Lyndon Johnson. The Urban Institute engages in policy analysis, program evaluation, and informing community development. The focus of the Urban Institute is to improve social, civic, and economic well-being. The mission of the Urban Institute is to gather data, conduct research, evaluate programs, conduct policy analysis, offer international technical assistance, and educate Americans regarding social and economic issues. The Urban Institute has eleven policy centers: assessing the New Federalism; education; health; income and benefits; international development and governance; justice; labor, human services, and population; low-income working families; metropolitan housing and communities; nonprofits and philanthropy; and Urban-Brookings tax.

Summary Points

- Policy institutes engage in activities such as policymaking, policy analysis, policy evaluation, and policy research.
- Policy institutes each have a focus area of interest.
- Policy institutes may be membership based, and/or have a group of experts and scholars who conduct the activities of the policy institute.
- The products of policy institutes include books, reports, briefs, testimony, educational materials, conferences, and seminars.

Presidential and Congressional Leadership: Political Party Leadership

Presidential leadership			Congressional leadership		
Time period	President	Political party	Congress	Majority party	Minority party
1789–1797	George Washington	Independent	1st (1789–1791)	Pro-administration	Anti-administration
			2nd (1791–1793)	Pro-administration	Anti-administration
			3rd (1793–1795)	Pro-administration	Anti-administration
			4th (1795–1797)	Federalist	Republican
1797–1801	John Adams	Federalist	5th (1797–1799)	Federalist	Republican
			6th (1799–1801)	Federalist	Republican
1801–1809	Thomas Jefferson	Democratic-Republican	7th (1801–1803)	Republican	Federalist
			8th (1803–1805)	Republican	Federalist
			9th (1805–1807)	Republican	Federalist
			10th (1807–1809)	Republican	Federalist
1809–1817	James Madison	Democratic-Republican	11th (1809–1811)	Republican	Federalist
			12th (1811–1813)	Republican	Federalist
			13th (1813–1815)	Republican	Federalist
			14th (1815–1817)	Republican	Federalist
1817–1825	James Monroe	Democratic-Republican	15th (1817–1819)	Republican	Federalist
			16th (1819–1821)	Republican	Federalist
			17th (1821–1823)	Republican	Federalist
			18th (1823–1825)	Republican	Federalist
1825–1829	John Q. Adams	Democratic-Republican National Republican	19th (1825–1827)	Jacksonian	Adams
			20th (1827–1829)	Jacksonian	Adams

Years	President	Party	Congress		
1829–1837	Andrew Jackson	Democratic	21st (1829–1831)	Jacksonian	Anti-Jackson
			22nd (1831–1833)	Jacksonian	Anti-Jackson
			23rd (1833–1835)	Anti-Jackson	Jackson
			24th (1835–1837)	Jacksonian	Anti-Jackson
1837–1841	Martin Van Buren	Democratic	25th (1837–1839)	Democratic	Whig
			26th (1839–1841)	Democratic	Whig
1841–1841	William H. Harrison	Whig	27th (1841–1843)	Whig	Democratic
1841–1845	John Tyler	Whig (1841–1841) Independent (1841–1845)	28th (1841–1845)	Whig	Democratic
1845–1849	James K. Polk	Democratic	29th (1845–1847)	Democratic	Whig
			30th (1847–1849)	Democratic	Whig
1849–1850	Zachary Taylor	Whig	31st (1849–1851)	Democratic	Whig
1850–1853	Millard Fillmore	Whig	32nd (1851–1853)	Democratic	Whig
1853–1857	Franklin Pierce	Democratic	33rd (1853–1855)	Democratic	Whig
			34th (1855–1857)	Democratic	Opposition
1857–1861	James Buchanan	Democratic	35th (1857–1859)	Democratic	Republican
			36th (1859–1861)	Democratic	Republican
1861–1865	Abraham Lincoln	Republican National Union	37th (1861–1863)	Republican	Democratic
			38th (1863–1865)	Republican	Democratic
1865–1869	Andrew Johnson	Democratic National Union and Independent	39th (1865–1867)	Republican	Democratic
			40th (1867–1869)	Republican	Democratic

(continues)

	Presidential leadership		Congressional leadership		
Time period	President	Political party	Congress	Majority party	Minority party
1869–1877	Ulysses S. Grant	Republican	41st (1869–1871)	Republican	Democratic
			42nd (1871–1873)	Republican	Democratic
			43rd (1873–1875)	Republican	Democratic
			44th (1875–1877)	Republican	Democratic
1877–1881	Rutherford B. Hayes	Republican	45th (1877–1879)	Republican	Democratic
			46th (1879–1881)	Democratic	Republican
1881–1881	James A. Garfield	Republican	47th (1881–1883)	Republican	Democratic
1881–1885	Chester A. Arthur	Republican	48th (1883–1885)	Republican	Democratic
1885–1889	Grover Cleveland	Democratic	49th (1885–1887)	Republican	Democratic
			50th (1887–1889)	Republican	Democratic
1889–1893	Benjamin Harrison	Republican	51st (1889–1891)	Republican	Democratic
			52nd (1891–1893)	Republican	Democratic
1893–1897	Grover Cleveland	Democratic	53rd (1893–1895)	Democratic	Republican
			54th (1895–1897)	Republican	Democratic
1897–1901	William McKinley	Republican	55th (1897–1899)	Republican	Democratic
			56th (1899–1901)	Republican	Democratic
1901–1909	Theodore Roosevelt	Republican	57th (1901–1903)	Republican	Democratic
			58th (1903–1905)	Republican	Democratic
			59th (1905–1907)	Republican	Democratic
			60th (1907–1909)	Republican	Democratic
1909–1913	William H. Taft	Republican	61st (1909–1911)	Republican	Democratic
			62nd (1911–1913)	Republican	Democratic

Years	President	President's Party	Congress	House	Senate
1913–1921	Woodrow Wilson	Democratic	63rd (1913–1915)	Democratic	Republican
			64th (1915–1917)	Democratic	Republican
			65th (1917–1919)	Democratic	Republican
			66th (1919–1921)	Republican	Democratic
1921–1923	Warren G. Harding	Republican	67th (1921–1923)	Republican	Republican
1923–1929	Calvin Coolidge	Republican	68th (1923–1925)	Republican	Democratic
			69th (1925–1927)	Republican	Democratic
			70th (1927–1929)	Republican	Democratic
1929–1933	Herbert Hoover	Republican	71st (1929–1931)	Republican	Democratic
			72nd (1931–1933)	Republican	Democratic
1933–1945	Franklin D. Roosevelt	Democratic	73rd (1933–1935)	Democratic	Democratic
			74th (1935–1937)	Democratic	Democratic
			75th (1937–1939)	Democratic	Democratic
			76th (1939–1941)	Democratic	Democratic
			77th (1941–1943)	Democratic	Democratic
			78th (1943–1945)	Democratic	Democratic
1945–1953	Harry S. Truman	Democratic	79th (1945–1947)	Democratic	Democratic
			80th (1947–1949)	Republican	Republican
			81st (1949–1951)	Democratic	Democratic
			82nd (1951–1953)	Democratic	Democratic
1953–1961	Dwight D. Eisenhower	Republican	83rd (1953–1955)	Republican	Democratic
			84th (1955–1957)	Democratic	Republican
			85th (1957–1959)	Democratic	Republican
			86th (1959–1961)	Democratic	Republican

(continues)

Presidential leadership			Congressional leadership		
Time period	President	Political party	Congress	Majority party	Minority party
1961–1963	John F. Kennedy	Democratic	87th (1961–1963)	Democratic	Republican
1963–1969	Lyndon B. Johnson	Democratic	88th (1963–1965)	Democratic	Republican
			89th (1965–1967)	Democratic	Republican
			90th (1967–1969)	Democratic	Republican
1969–1974	Richard Nixon	Republican	91st (1969–1971)	Democratic	Republican
			92nd (1971–1973)	Democratic	Republican
			93rd (1973–1975)	Democratic	Republican
1974–1977	Gerald Ford	Republican	94th (1975–1977)	Democratic	Republican
1977–1981	Jimmy Carter	Democratic	95th (1977–1979)	Democratic	Republican
			96th (1979–1981)	Democratic	Republican
1981–1989	Ronald Reagan	Republican	97th (1981–1983)	Republican	Democratic
			98th (1983–1985)	Republican	Democratic
			99th (1985–1987)	Republican	Democratic
			100th (1987–1989)	Democratic	Republican
1989–1993	George H.W. Bush	Republican	101st (1989–1991)	Democratic	Republican
			102nd (1991–1993)	Democratic	Republican
1993–2001	Bill Clinton	Democratic	103rd (1993–1995)	Democratic	Republican
			104th (1995–1997)	Republican	Democratic
			105th (1997–1999)	Republican	Democratic
			106th (1999–2001)	Republican	Democratic

		107th (2001–2003)	Democratic then	Republican, then
2001–2009	George W. Bush	Republican	Republican, then	Democratic, then
			Democratic, then	Republican, then
		108th (2003–2005)	Republican	Democratic
		109th (2005–2007)	Republican	Democratic
		110th (2007–2009)	Democratic	Democratic
				Republican
2009–Present	Barack Obama	Democratic		
		111th (2009–2011)	Democratic	Republican
		112th (2011–2013)	Republican	Democratic

Note: Presidency is defined as a consecutive time in office. Congress is defined as the time in which the House of Representatives get a new term of office.

List of Public Laws*

Congress of the Confederation

1. Northwest Ordinance of 1784
2. Land Ordinance of 1785

1st US Congress

1. Act to regulate time and manner of administering certain oaths
2. Hamilton Tariff
3. Judiciary Act of 1789
4. Census of 1790
5. Naturalization Act of 1790
6. Patent Act
7. Southwest Ordinance
8. Copyright Act of 1790
9. Residence Act
10. Indian Intercourse Act of 1790
11. First Bank of the United States
12. Whiskey Act

*The public laws list is not comprehensive. Public and private public laws can be located and accessed through the Office of the Federal Register online at http://www.gpoaccess.gov/nara/index.html.

2nd US Congress

1. Postal Service Act
2. Coinage Act of 1792
3. First Militia Act of 1792
4. Second Militia Act of 1792
5. Fugitive Slave Law of 1793
6. Judiciary Act of 1793 (including Anti-Injunction Act)

3rd US Congress

1. Naval Act of 1794
2. Naturalization Act of 1795

4th US Congress

1. Treaty of Madrid

5th US Congress

1. The US Department of the Navy was established
2. Alien and Sedition Acts to establish a uniform rule of naturalization (Naturalization Act of 1798)
3. The Marine Corps was established
4. Alien and Sedition Acts for the punishment of certain crimes against the United States (Sedition Acts)

6th US Congress

1. Judiciary Act of 1801
2. District of Columbia Organic Act of 1801

7th US Congress

1. Judiciary Act of 1802
2. Enabling Act of 1802

8th US Congress

1. Louisiana Purchase

9th US Congress

10th US Congress

1. Embargo Act of 1807
2. Non-Intercourse Act

11th US Congress

    1. Macon's Bill Number 2

12th US Congress

    1. Declaration of War on Great Britain

13th US Congress

    1. Treaty of Ghent

14th US Congress

    1. Second Bank of the United States

15th US Congress

    1. Flag Act of 1818
    2. Navigation Act of 1818

16th US Congress

    1. Land Act of 1820

17th US Congress

18th US Congress

    1. Tariff of 1824

19th US Congress

    1. Treaty of Washington

20th US Congress

    1. Tariff of Abominations

21st US Congress

    1. Indian Removal Act

22nd US Congress

    1. Tariff of 1832
    2. Compromise Tariff (Tariff of 1833)
    3. Force Bill

23rd US Congress

24th US Congress

25th US Congress

26th US Congress

27th US Congress

1. Bankruptcy Act of 1841
2. Preemption Act of 1841
3. Tariff of 1842 ("Black Tariff")

28th US Congress

29th US Congress

1. District of Columbia retrocession
2. Walker tariff

30th US Congress

1. Coinage Act of 1849

31st US Congress

1. Fugitive Slave Act
2. Donation Land Claim Act

32nd US Congress

33rd US Congress

1. Kansas-Nebraska Act

34th US Congress

1. Guano Islands Act

35th US Congress

36th US Congress

1. Morrill Tariff

37th US Congress

1. Revenue Act of 1861
2. Confiscation Act of 1861
3. Legal Tender Act of 1862

4. Homestead Act
5. Morrill Anti-Bigamy Act
6. Revenue Act of 1862
7. Pacific Railway Act
8. Morrill Land Grant Colleges Act
9. Militia Act
10. National Banking Act
11. False Claims Act
12. Enrollment Act

38th US Congress

1. Coinage Act of 1864

39th US Congress

1. Civil Rights Act of 1866
2. Judicial Circuits Act
3. Reconstruction Act
4. Tenure of Office Act

40th US Congress

1. Reconstruction Acts

41st US Congress

1. Judiciary Act of 1869 (Circuit Judges Act of 1869)
2. Force Act of 1870
3. Naturalization Act of 1870
4. District of Columbia Organic Act of 1871

42nd US Congress

1. Ku Klux Act (Civil Rights Act of 1871, Ku Klux Klan Act)
2. Yellowstone Act
3. General Mining Act of 1872
4. Amnesty Act
5. Practice Conformity Act (precursor to the Rules Enabling Act)
6. Coinage Act of 1873
7. Timber Culture Act

43rd US Congress

1. Civil Rights Act of 1875

44th US Congress

1. Desert Land Act

45th US Congress

1. Bland-Allison Act (Coinage Act [Silver Dollar])
2. National Quarantine Act
3. Timber and Stone Act

46th US Congress

47th US Congress

1. Chinese Exclusion Act
2. Pendleton Civil Service Reform Act

48th US Congress

49th US Congress

1. Interstate Commerce Act
2. Indian General Allotment Act (Dawes Act)
3. Hatch Act of 1887
4. Tucker Act
5. Edmunds-Tucker Act

50th US Congress

1. Enabling Act of 1889

51st US Congress

1. Sherman Antitrust Act
2. Sherman Silver Purchase Act
3. Morrill Land Grant College Act of 1890
4. McKinley Tariff
5. Forest Reserve Act of 1891
6. Land Revision Act of 1891

52nd US Congress

1. Geary Act (amended the Chinese Exclusion Act)

53rd US Congress

1. Wilson-Gorman Tariff Act
2. Maguire Act of 1895

54th US Congress

55th US Congress

1. Dingley Tariff (amended the Wilson-Gorman Tariff Act)
2. Bankruptcy Act of 1898
3. Newlands Resolution, No. 55
4. Rivers and Harbors Act of 1899

56th US Congress

1. Gold Standard Act
2. Foraker Act (Puerto Rico Civil Code)
3. Anarchist Exclusion Act

57th US Congress

1. Newlands Reclamation Act (National Irrigation Act, Reclamation Act)
2. Isthmian Canal Act (Panama Canal)
3. Militia Act of 1903 (Dick Act)

58th US Congress

1. Kinkaid Act

59th US Congress

1. Federal Employers' Liability Act
2. American Antiquities Act (National Monument Act)
3. Pure Food and Drug Act
4. Meat Inspection Act

60th US Congress

1. Aldrich-Vreeland Act

61st US Congress

1. Payne-Aldrich Tariff Act

62nd US Congress

1. Lloyd-La Follette Act

63rd US Congress

1. Revenue Act of 1913 (including Underwood Tariff)
2. Federal Reserve Act

3. Federal Trade Commission Act
4. Clayton Antitrust Act
5. Harrison Narcotics Tax Act

64th US Congress

1. Federal Farm Loan Act
2. National Park Service Act
3. Keating-Owen Child Labor Act of 1916
4. Revenue Act of 1916
5. Stock-Raising Homestead Act
6. Immigration Act of 1917 (Barred Zone Act)
7. Smith-Hughes Vocational Education Act
8. Flood Control Act of 1917

65th US Congress

1. 1st Liberty Loan Act
2. Enemy Vessel Confiscation Joint Resolution
3. 1st Army Appropriations Act of 1917
4. Selective Service Act of 1917
5. 2nd Army Appropriations Act of 1917
6. Search Warrant Act of 1917
7. Emergency Shipping Fund Act of 1917
8. Espionage Act of 1917
9. River and Harbors Act of 1917
10. Priority of Shipments Act of 1917
11. Obstruction of Interstate Commerce Act of 1917
12. Food and Fuel Control Act (Lever Act)
13. Grain Standards Act of 1917
14. 2nd Liberty Loan Act
15. Aircraft Board Act of 1917
16. War Revenue Act of 1917
17. Repatriation Act of 1917
18. Explosives Act of 1917
19. International Emergency Economic Powers Act (Trading with the Enemy Act)
20. War Risk Insurance Act of 1917
21. Smoot Amendment
22. Federal Possession and Control Act
23. Revenue Act of 1918

24. Soldiers' and Sailors' Civil Relief Act
25. Standard Time Act (Calder Act)
26. Daylight Savings Act (Borland-Calder Act)
27. Federal Control Act of 1918
28. 3rd Liberty Loan Act
29. War Finance Corporation Act
30. American Forces Abroad Indemnity Act
31. Destruction of War Materials Act
32. Alien Naturalization Act
33. Housing for War Needs Act
34. Departmental Reorganization Act (Overman Act)
35. Passport Control Act
36. Entry and Departure Controls Act
37. Veterans Rehabilitation Act (Smith-Sears Act)
38. Industrial Aid Act (Fess Act)
39. Migratory Bird Treaty Act of 1918
40. Army Appropriations Act of 1918
41. 4th Liberty Loan Act
42. Public Health and Research Act of 1918 (Chamberlain-Kahn Act)
43. Charter Rate and Requisition Act of 1918
44. River and Harbors Act of 1918
45. Immigration Act of October 16, 1918 (Dillingham-Hardwick Act)
46. Corrupt Practices Act of 1918 (Gerry Act)
47. National Bank Consolidation Act of 1918
48. War-Time Prohibition Act
49. Revenue Act of 1919
50. Child Labor Act of 1919
51. Grand Canyon Park Act of 1919
52. Acadia National Park Act of 1919
53. River and Harbors Act of 1919
54. War Minerals Relief Act of 1919 (Dent Act)
55. Hospitalization Act of 1919
56. War Risk Insurance Act of 1919
57. 5th Liberty Loan Act
58. Wheat Price Guarantee Act (Lever Act)

66th US Congress

1. National Prohibition Act (Volstead Act)
2. Mineral Leasing Act

67th US Congress

1. Emergency Quota Act (Johnson Quota Act)
2. Emergency Tariff of 1921
3. Future Trading Act
4. Revenue Act of 1921
5. Fordney-McCumber tariff
6. Grain Futures Act
7. Cable Act (Married Women's Citizenship Act)

68th US Congress

1. World War Adjusted Compensation Act (Bonus Bill)
2. Immigration Act of 1924 (Johnson-Reed Act)
3. Indian Citizenship Act of 1924 (Snyder Act)
4. Revenue Act of 1924 (Mellon tax bill)

69th US Congress

1. Revenue Act of 1926

70th US Congress

1. Settlement of War Claims Act
2. Flood Control Act of 1928 (Jones-Reid Act)
3. Merchant Marine Act of 1928 (Jones-White Act)
4. Forest Research Act (McSweeney-McNary Act)
5. Revenue Act of 1928
6. Boulder Canyon Project Act (Hoover Dam)
7. Color of Title Act
8. Migratory Bird Conservation Act (Norbeck-Anderson Act)
9. Increased Penalties Act (Jones-Stalker Act)

71st US Congress

1. Migratory Bird Conservation Act
2. Agriculture Marketing Act
3. Reapportionment Act of 1929
4. Hawley-Smoot Tariff (including Plant Patent Act)

72nd US Congress

1. Reconstruction Finance Corporation Act
2. Revenue Act of 1932

3. Federal Home Loan Bank Act
4. Buy American Act

73rd US Congress

1. Emergency Banking Relief Act
2. Economy Act
3. Civilian Conservation Corps Reforestation Relief Act
4. Federal Emergency Relief Act
5. Agricultural Adjustment Act
6. Securities Act
7. Home Owners' Loan Corporation
8. Glass-Steagall Act (Banking Act of 1933)
9. National Industrial Recovery Act
10. Farm Credit Administration
11. Tydings-McDuffie Act (Philippine Independence Act)
12. Johnson Act
13. Securities Exchange Act
14. Reciprocal Tariff Act
15. Indian Reorganization Act
16. Rules Enabling Act
17. Communications Act of 1934
18. National Archives Act
19. Federal Credit Union Act
20. National Firearms Act of 1934
21. National Housing Act (including Federal National Mortgage Association Charter Act/Fannie Mae)

74th US Congress

1. Soil Conservation and Domestic Allotment Act
2. National Labor Relations Act (Wagner Act)
3. Motor Carrier Act (renamed part II of the Interstate Commerce Act)
4. Social Security Act (including Aid to Dependent Children, Old Age Pension Act)
5. Public Utility Act (including: Public Utility Holding Company Act of 1935, Federal Power Act)
6. Revenue Act of 1935
7. Neutrality Act of 1935
8. Neutrality Act of 1936
9. Rural Electrification Act

10. Commodities Exchange Act
11. Flood Control Act of 1936
12. Merchant Marine Act
13. Walsh-Healey Public Contracts Act

75th US Congress

1. Agricultural Marketing Agreement Act
2. Marijuana Tax Act
3. National Cancer Institute Act
4. 1937: Neutrality Acts of 1937
5. Foreign Agents Registration Act
6. Natural Gas Act
7. Civil Aeronautics Act
8. Fair Labor Standards Act
9. Federal Food, Drug, and Cosmetic Act

76th US Congress

1. Reorganization Act of 1939
2. Hatch Act of 1939 (Hatch Political Activity Act, An Act to Prevent Pernicious Political Activities)
3. Neutrality Act of 1939, (Cash and Carry Act)
4. Investment Company Act of 1940
5. Investment Advisers Act of 1940
6. Alien Registration Act (Smith Act)
7. Selective Training and Service Act of 1940
8. Investment Company Act of 1940

77th US Congress

1. Lend Lease Act
2. Flood Control Act of 1941
3. Emergency Price Control Act

78th US Congress

1. Magnuson Act (Chinese Exclusion Repeal Act of 1943)
2. Mustering-out Payment Act
3. Servicemen's Readjustment Act of 1944 (G.I. Bill)
4. Veterans' Preference Act
5. Public Health Service Act
6. Pick-Sloan Flood Control Act

79th US Congress

1. Export-Import Bank Act of 1945
2. United Nations Participation Act
3. War Brides Act
4. Rescission Act of 1946
5. Employment Act
6. Federal Airport Act
7. Richard B. Russell National School Lunch Act
8. Administrative Procedure Act
9. Hobbs Anti-Racketeering Act
10. Lanham Trademark Act of 1946
11. United States Atomic Energy Act of 1946
12. Legislative Reorganization Act of 1946
13. Federal Tort Claims Act
14. Federal Regulation of Lobbying Act of 1946
15. Foreign Service Act
16. Hospital Survey and Construction Act (Hill-Burton Act)
17. Farmers Home Administration Act

80th US Congress

1. National Security Act of 1947
2. Mineral Leasing Act for Acquired Lands
3. United States Information and Educational Exchange Act
4. Foreign Assistance Act (Marshall Plan)
5. Greek-Turkish Assistance Act of 1948
6. Civil Air Patrol Act
7. Presidential Succession Act
8. Federal Water Pollution Control Act
9. War Claims Act of 1948

81st US Congress

1. Central Intelligence Agency Act
2. Uniform Code of Military Justice
3. National Science Foundation Act
4. McCarran Internal Security Act
5. Federal Civil Defense Act of 1950

82nd US Congress

1. Mutual Security Act
2. Immigration and Nationality Act (McCarran-Walter Act)

3. Veterans' Readjustment Assistance Act
4. Federal Coal Mine Safety Act Amendments of 1952

83rd US Congress

1. Small Business Act
2. Refugee Relief Act
3. Outer Continental Shelf Lands Act
4. Federal National Mortgage Association Charter Act
5. Multiple Mineral Development Act
6. Internal Revenue Code of 1954
7. Federal Unemployment Tax Act
8. National Firearms Act
9. Communist Control Act of 1954

84th US Congress

1. Flood Control and Coastal Emergency Act
2. Air Pollution Control Act
3. Poliomyelitis Vaccination Assistance Act
4. Health Research Facilities Act
5. Federal-Aid Highway Act of 1956 (National Interstate and Defense Highways Act)

85th US Congress

1. Airways Modernization Act
2. Price-Anderson Nuclear Industries Indemnity Act
3. Civil Rights Act of 1957
4. National Aeronautics and Space Act
5. Transportation Act of 1958
6. Federal Aviation Act
7. Military Construction Appropriation Act (Advanced Research Projects Agency)
8. National Defense Education Act
9. Department of Defense Reorganization Act

86th US Congress

1. Admission of Hawaii Act
2. Airport Construction Act
3. Landrum-Griffin Act
4. Civil Rights Act of 1960

5. Social Security Amendments (Kerr-Mill aid)
6. Flood Control Act of 1960

87th US Congress

1. Area Redevelopment Act
2. Foreign Assistance Act of 1961
3. Interstate Wire Act of 1961
4. Mutual Educational and Cultural Exchange Act of 1961
5. Peace Corps Act of 1961
6. Arms Control and Disarmament Act
7. Community Health Services and Facilities Act
8. Manpower Development and Training Act
9. Migration and Refugee Assistance Act
10. Communications Satellite Act of 1962
11. Trade Expansion Act
12. Bribery Act
13. Vaccination Assistance Act
14. Rivers and Harbors Act of 1962

88th US Congress

1. Equal Pay Act
2. Community Mental Health Centers Act (including Mental Retardation Facilities Construction Act)
3. Clean Air Act
4. Civil Rights Act of 1964
5. Urban Mass Transportation Act of 1964 (Federal Transit Act)
6. Economic Opportunity Act of 1964
7. Food Stamp Act of 1964
8. Wilderness Act
9. Land and Water Conservation Act
10. Nurse Training Act

89th US Congress

1. Elementary and Secondary Education Act
2. Federal Cigarette Labeling and Advertising Act
3. Social Security Act of 1965 (including Medicaid and Medicare)
4. Voting Rights Act
5. Housing and Urban Development Act of 1965
6. Public Works and Economic Development Act of 1965

7. National Foundation on the Arts and the Humanities Act
8. Immigration and Nationality Act of 1965
9. Heart Disease, Cancer, and Stroke Amendments
10. Motor Vehicle Air Pollution Control Act (including Solid Waste Disposal Act)
11. Highway Beautification Act
12. Higher Education Act
13. Vocational Rehabilitation Act Amendments
14. Uniform Time Act
15. Freedom of Information Act
16. National Traffic and Motor Vehicle Safety Act
17. National Historic Preservation Act
18. National Wildlife Refuge System Administration Act
19. Department of Transportation Act
20. Cuban Adjustment Act
21. Comprehensive Health, Planning, and Service Act

90th US Congress

1. Supplemental Defense Appropriations Act
2. Public Broadcasting Act
3. Age Discrimination in Employment Act
4. National Park Foundation Act
5. Bilingual Education Act
6. Civil Rights Act of 1968
7. Consumer Cr Protection Act
8. Omnibus Crime Control and Safe Streets Act of 1968
9. Uniform Monday Holiday Act
10. Aircraft Noise Abatement Act
11. Architectural Barriers Act of 1968
12. Wild and Scenic Rivers Act
13. National Trails System Act
14. Gun Control Act of 1968

91st US Congress

1. Federal Coal Mine Health and Safety Act
2. Truth in Lending Act
3. National Environmental Policy Act
4. Airport and Airway Development Act
5. District of Columbia Delegate Act

6. Organized Crime Control Act (including the Racketeer Influenced and Corrupt Organizations Act [RICO])
7. Bank Secrecy Act
8. Controlled Substances Act
9. Postal Reorganization Act (United States Postal Service)
10. Urban Mass Transportation Act of 1970
11. Rail Passenger Service Act (Amtrak)
12. Family Planning Services and Population Research Act of 1970
13. Plant Variety Protection Act
14. Occupational Safety and Health Act (OSHA)
15. Clean Air Act Extension
16. Housing and Urban Development Act of 1970 (including National Urban Policy and New Community Development Act of 1970)
17. Lead-Based Paint Poisoning Prevention Act
18. Economic Stabilization Act
19. Environmental Quality Improvement Act

92nd US Congress

1. Alaska Native Claims Settlement Act
2. National Cancer Act
3. Federal Election Campaign Act
4. Equal Employment Opportunity Act
5. Title IX Amendment of the Higher Education Act
6. Federal Advisory Committee Act
7. Federal Water Pollution Control Amendments of 1972
8. Marine Mammal Protection Act
9. Marine Protection, Research and Sanctuaries Act
10. Consumer Product Safety Act
11. Noise Control Act
12. Coastal Zone Management Act

93rd US Congress

1. Federal Aid Highway Act of 1973
2. Rehabilitation Act
3. Domestic Volunteer Services Act of 1973 (VISTA)
4. Amtrak Improvement Act
5. War Powers Resolution
6. District of Columbia Home Rule Act
7. Comprehensive Employment and Training Act

8. Endangered Species Act
9. Water Resources Development Act of 1974
10. Disaster Relief Act of 1974
11. Research on Aging Act
12. Congressional Budget and Impoundment Control Act of 1974
13. Legal Services Corporation Act
14. Family Educational Rights and Privacy Act
15. Employee Retirement Income Security Act (ERISA)
16. Juvenile Justice and Delinquency Prevention Act of 1974
17. National Mass Transportation Assistance Act
18. Vietnam Era Veterans' Readjustment Assistance Act
19. Safe Drinking Water Act
20. Privacy Act of 1974
21. Trade Act of 1974
22. Federal Noxious Weed Act of 1974
23. Hazardous Materials Transportation Act
24. National Health Planning and Resources Development Act

94th US Congress

1. Revenue Adjustment Act (Earned Income Tax Credit)
2. Individuals with Disabilities Education Act
3. Railroad Revitalization and Regulatory Reform Act
4. Government in the Sunshine Act
5. Hart-Scott-Rodino Antitrust Improvements Act
6. Toxic Substances Control Act
7. Overhaul of vocational education programs
8. Copyright Act of 1976
9. Federal Land Policy and Management Act
10. Resource Conservation and Recovery Act
11. Water Resources Development Act of 1976
12. National Forest Management Act

95th US Congress

1. Surface Mining Control and Reclamation Act
2. Community Reinvestment Act
3. Unlawful Corporate Payments Act of 1977 (including Foreign Corrupt Practices Act)
4. Clean Water Act

5. International Emergency Economic Powers Act
6. Department of Energy Organization Act
7. Nuclear Non-Proliferation Act
8. Civil Service Reform Act
9. Drug Abuse Prevention, Treatment, and Rehabilitation Act
10. Airline Deregulation Act
11. Foreign Intelligence Surveillance Act
12. Ethics in Government Act
13. Humphrey-Hawkins Full Employment Act
14. Pregnancy Discrimination Act
15. Contract Disputes Act
16. Bankruptcy Act of 1978
17. Public Utility Regulatory Policies Act
18. National Energy Conservation Policy Act

96th US Congress

1. Panama Canal Act of 1979
2. Department of Education Organization Act
3. Refugee Act
4. Regulatory Flexibility Act
5. Fish and Wildlife Conservation Act of 1980
6. Alaska National Interest Lands Conservation Act
7. Comprehensive Environmental Response, Compensation, and Liability Act (CERCLA or Superfund)
8. Paperwork Reduction Act of 1980

97th US Congress

1. Economic Recovery Tax Act (ERTA or Kemp-Roth Tax Cut)
2. Omnibus Budget Reconciliation Act of 1981
3. Bus Regulatory Reform Act
4. Job Training Partnership Act
5. Garn-St Germain Depository Institutions Act
6. Surface Transportation Assistance Act
7. Nuclear Waste Policy Act

98th US Congress

1. Voting Accessibility for the Elderly and Handicapped Act
2. Comprehensive Crime Control Act

99th US Congress

1. Balanced Budget and Emergency Deficit Control Act of 1985 (Gramm-Rudman-Hollings Balanced Budget Act)
2. Gold Bullion Coin Act of 1985
3. Consolidated Omnibus Budget Reconciliation Act of 1985 (COBRA) (including Emergency Medical Treatment and Active Labor Act)
4. Goldwater-Nichols Act of 1986 (Defense Reorganization)
5. Comprehensive Anti-Apartheid Act
6. Immigration Reform and Control Act of 1986 (Simpson-Mazzoli Act)
7. Emergency Planning and Community Right-to-Know Act (title III)
8. Electronic Communications Privacy Act of 1986
9. Tax Reform Act of 1986
10. Anti-Drug Abuse Act
11. Age Discrimination in Employment Act
12. Water Resources Development Act of 1986

100th US Congress

1. Surface Transportation and Uniform Relocation Assistance Act
2. Malcolm Baldrige National Quality Improvement Act of 1987
3. Balanced Budget and Emergency Deficit Control Reaffirmation Act of 1987 (Gramm-Rudman-Hollings Balanced Budget Act)
4. Agricultural Credit Act of 1987
5. Computer Security Act of 1987
6. Medicare Catastrophic Coverage Act
7. Civil Liberties Act
8. Family Support Act
9. Indian Gaming Regulatory Act
10. Department of Veterans Affairs Act
11. Water Resources Development Act of 1988
12. Anti-Drug Abuse Act of 1988 (including Child Protection and Obscenity Enforcement Act, Alcoholic Beverage Labeling Act)

101st US Congress

1. Whistleblower Protection Act
2. Water Resources Development Act 1990
3. Flag Protection Act of 1989
4. Americans with Disabilities Act

5. Omnibus Budget Reconciliation Act of 1990 (including Human Genome Project funding)
6. Water Resources Development Act of 1990
7. Administrative Dispute Resolution Act
8. Native American Graves Protection and Repatriation Act
9. Negotiated Rulemaking Act
10. Immigration Act of 1990
11. Judicial Improvements Act of 1990 (including Visual Artists Rights Act)

102nd US Congress

1. Civil Rights Act of 1991
2. High Performance Computing and Communication Act of 1991
3. Intermodal Surface Transportation Efficiency Act
4. Chinese Student Protection Act of 1992
5. Weapons of Mass Destruction Control Act
6. Water Resources Development Act of 1992

103rd US Congress

1. Family and Medical Leave Act
2. National Voter Registration Act of 1993
3. Omnibus Budget Reconciliation Act of 1993
4. Religious Freedom Restoration Act
5. Brady Handgun Violence Prevention Act (Brady Bill)
6. National Defense Authorization Act for Fiscal Year 1994 (including "Don't Ask, Don't Tell")
7. North American Free Trade Agreement Implementation Act
8. Freedom of Access to Clinic Entrances Act
9. Violent Crime Control and Law Enforcement Act (including the Violence Against Women Act)

104th US Congress

1. Congressional Accountability Act
2. National Highway Designation Act
3. Lobbying Disclosure Act
4. Private Securities Litigation Reform Act
5. Telecommunications Act of 1996 (including the Communications Decency Act)

6. Cuban Liberty and Democratic Solidarity (Libertad) Act of 1996 (Helms-Burton Act)
7. Line Item Veto Act
8. Antiterrorism and Effective Death Penalty Act
9. Taxpayer Bill of Rights 2
10. National Gambling Impact Study Commission Act
11. Small Business Job Protection Act
12. Health Insurance Portability and Accountability Act (HIPAA)
13. Personal Responsibility and Work Opportunity Act (Welfare Reform Act)
14. Defense of Marriage Act
15. Domestic Violence Offender Gun Ban
16. Emerson Good Samaritan Food Donation Act
17. Water Resources Development Act of 1996

105th US Congress

1. Balanced Budget Act of 1997
2. Taxpayer Relief Act of 1997
3. Transportation Equity Act for the 21st Century
4. Taxpayer Bill of Rights III
5. Workforce Investment Act
6. Child Online Privacy Protection Act
7. Sonny Bono Copyright Term Extension Act
8. Digital Millennium Copyright Act (including Online Copyright Infringement Liability Limitation Act)
9. Iraq Liberation Act

106th US Congress

1. Emergency Supplemental Appropriations Act (Kosovo operations)
2. Water Resources Development Act of 1999
3. Gramm-Leach-Bliley Financial Services Modernization Act
4. American Inventors Protection Act (including Anticybersquatting Consumer Protection Act)
5. Iran Nonproliferation Act of 2000
6. Wendell H. Ford Aviation Investment and Reform Act for the 21st Century
7. African Growth and Opportunity Act
8. Electronic Signatures in Global and National Commerce Act

9. Oceans Act
10. Religious Land Use and Institutionalized Persons Act
11. Children's Health Act
12. Robert T. Stafford Disaster Relief and Emergency Assistance Act
13. Water Resources Development Act of 2000
14. Commodity Futures Modernization Act of 2000 (as part of the Consolidated Appropriations Act, 2001)

107th US Congress

1. Economic Growth and Tax Relief Reconciliation Act
2. Uniting and Strengthening America by Providing Appropriate Tools Required to Intercept and Obstruct Terrorism (USA PATRIOT) Act
3. No Child Left Behind Act
4. Small Business Liability Relief and Brownfields Revitalization Act
5. Job Creation and Worker Assistance Act
6. Bipartisan Campaign Reform Act (McCain-Feingold)
7. Farm Security and Rural Investment Act of 2002
8. Sarbanes-Oxley Act
9. Trade Act of 2002
10. Authorization for Use of Military Force Against Iraq
11. Sudan Peace Act
12. Help America Vote Act
13. Homeland Security Act
14. E-Government Act of 2002

108th US Congress

1. Do-Not-Call Implementation Act of 2003
2. PROTECT (Prosecutorial Remedies and Other Tools to end the Exploitation of Children Today) Act (including Illicit Drug Anti-Proliferation Act)
3. Jobs and Growth Tax Relief Reconciliation Act of 2003
4. Prison Rape Elimination Act of 2003
5. Partial-Birth Abortion Ban Act
6. Medicare Prescription Drug, Improvement, and Modernization Act
7. Fair and Accurate Credit Transactions Act
8. Syria Accountability and Lebanese Sovereignty Restoration Act
9. CAN-SPAM Act
10. Unborn Victims of Violence Act (Laci and Conner's Law)

11. Bunning-Bereuter-Blumenauer Flood Insurance Reform Act
12. GAO Human Capital Reform Act of 2004
13. Global Anti-Semitism Review Act
14. North Korean Human Rights Act of 2004
15. Belarus Democracy Act of 2004
16. Intelligence Reform and Terrorism Prevention Act

109th US Congress

1. Class Action Fairness Act of 2005
2. Bankruptcy Abuse Prevention and Consumer Protection Act
3. Family Entertainment and Copyright Act
4. Dominican Republic-Central America-United States Free Trade Agreement Implementation Act (CAFTA Implementation Act)
5. Energy Policy Act of 2005
6. Transportation Equity Act of 2005
7. Protection of Lawful Commerce in Arms Act
8. Caribbean National Forest Act of 2005
9. Department of Defense Appropriations Act (including McCain Detainee Amendment)
10. Deficit Reduction Act of 2005 (including Federal Deposit Insurance Reform Act)
11. Tax Increase Prevention and Reconciliation Act of 2005
12. Respect for America's Fallen Heroes Act
13. Adam Walsh Child Protection and Safety Act
14. Federal Funding Accountability and Transparency Act of 2006
15. Safe Port Act (including Unlawful Internet Gambling Enforcement Act of 2006)
16. Military Commissions Act of 2006
17. Secure Fence Act of 2006
18. Combating Autism Act
19. Tax Relief and Health Act of 2006

110th US Congress

1. House Page Board Revision Act of 2007
2. US Troop Readiness, Veterans' Care, Katrina Recovery, and Iraq Accountability Appropriations Act of 2007
3. Preserving United States Attorney Independence Act of 2007 (including Fair Minimum Wage Act of 2007)
4. Foreign Investment and National Security Act of 2007

5. Implementing Recommendations of the 9/11 Commission Act of 2007
6. Protect America Act of 2007
7. Honest Leadership and Open Government Act
8. Water Resources Development Act of 2007
9. Energy Independence and Security Act of 2007
10. Economic Stimulus Act of 2008
11. Genetic Information Nondiscrimination Act
12. Food and Energy Security Act of 2007 (2007 Farm Bill)
13. Supplemental Appropriations Act of 2008 (including Post-9/11 Veterans Educational Assistance Act of 2008/G.I. Bill 2008)
14. FISA Amendments Act of 2008
15. Housing and Economic Recovery Act of 2008
16. Emergency Economic Stabilization Act of 2008

111th US Congress

1. Lilly Ledbetter Fair Pay Act of 2009
2. Children's Health Insurance Program Reauthorization Act (SCHIP)
3. American Recovery and Reinvestment Act of 2009 (ARRA)
4. Omnibus Appropriations Act of 2009
5. Omnibus Public Land Management Act
6. Edward M. Kennedy Serve America Act
7. Fraud Enforcement and Recovery Act of 2009 (FERA)
8. Helping Families Save Their Homes Act of 2009
9. Weapon Systems Acquisition Reform Act of 2009
10. Family Smoking Prevention and Tobacco Control Act
11. Supplemental Appropriations Act of 2009
12. National Defense Authorization Act for Fiscal Year 2010, including the Matthew Shepard and James Byrd, Jr. Hate Crimes Prevention Act
13. Worker, Homeownership, and Business Assistance Act
14. Statutory Pay-As-You-Go Act
15. Patient Protection and Affordable Care Act

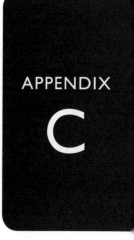

Policy Resources

Websites

Governmental Agencies and Centers

Administration for Children and Families: http://www.acf.hhs.gov

Administration on Aging (AoA): http://www.aoa.gov

Agency for HealthCare Research and Quality (AHRQ): http://www.ahrq.gov

American Association of Nurse Attorneys: http://www.taana.org

American Bar Association, health law section:
   http://www.abanet.org/health/home.html

American Health Lawyers Association: http://www.healthlawyers.org

American Society of Law, Medicine, and Ethics (ASLME):
   http://www.aslme.org

Bureau of Labor Statistics: http://www.bls.gov

Centers for Disease Control and Prevention (CDC): http://www.cdc.gov

Centers for Medicare and Medicaid Services: http://www.cms.gov

Chronic Disease Prevention and Health Promotion (of the CDC):
http://www.cdc.gov/chronicdisease

ClinicalTrials.gov: http://clinicaltrials.gov

Department of Health & Human Services: http://www.hhs.gov

Department of Veterans Affairs, health care section:
http://www1.va.gov/health

Government Accountability Office (GAO): http://www.gao.gov

Global Health Center (of the CDC): http://www.cdc.gov/globalhealth

Healthy People 2010: http://www.healthypeople.gov

Health Resources and Services Administration (HRSA): http://www.hrsa.gov

National Cancer Institute: http://www.cancer.gov

National Center for Complementary and Alternative Medicine (NCCAM):
http://www.nccam.nih.gov

National Center for Environmental Health (NCEH) (of the CDC):
http://www.cdc.gov/nceh

National Center for Health Statistics (of the CDC): http://www.cdc.gov/nchs

The National Center for Preparedness, Detection, and Control of Infectious
Diseases (NCPDCID) (of the CDC): http://www.cdc.gov/ncpdcid

National Health Law Program (NheLP): http://www.healthlaw.org

National Institute for Occupational Safety and Health (NIOSH) (of the CDC):
http://www.cdc.gov/niosh

National Center for Injury Prevention and Control (of the CDC):
http://www.cdc.gov/ncipc/ncipchm.htm

National Guideline Clearinghouse (of the AHRQ): http://www.guideline.gov

National Institutes of Health (NIH): http://www.nih.gov

National Library of Medicine (of the NIH): http://www.nlm.nih.gov

Occupational Safety & Health Administration (OSHA): http://osha.gov

Office of Disease Prevention and Health Promotion (ODPHP): http://www.healthfinder.gov

State Children's Health Insurance Program (SCHIP), FirstStep program: http://www.cms.gov/apps/firststep/content/schip-qas.html

US Congressional Budget Office (CBO): http://www.cbo.gov

US Food and Drug Administration (FDA): http://www.fda.gov

Associations and Professional Organizations

The Alliance: http://www.the-alliance.org

American Academy of Family Physicians: http://familydoctor.org/online/famdocen/home.html

America's Health Insurance Plans (AHIP): http://www.ahip.org

American Association of Retired Persons (AARP): http://www.aarp.org/health

American Board of Medical Specialties (ABMS), CertiFACTS: http://www.certifacts.org

American Cancer Society: http://www.cancer.org

American College of Preventive Medicine (ACPM): http://www.acpm.org

American Health Care Association (AHCA): http://www.ahcancal.org

American Heart Association (AHA): http://www.heart.org

American Lung Association: http://www.lungusa.org

American Medical Association (AMA): http://www.ama-assn.org

American Public Health Association (APHA): http://www.apha.org

Annals of Long Term Care (American Geriatrics Society):
  http://www.annalsoflongtermcare.com

The Commonwealth Fund: http://www.commonwealthfund.org

Families USA: http://www.familiesusa.org

HealthCareCoach.com (National Health Law Program):
  http://www.healthcarecoach.com

Health Care Jobs Career Center: http://www.healthcarejobs.org

Joint Commission, accreditation programs section:
  http://www.jointcommission.org/AccreditationPrograms

Kaiser Family Foundation: http://www.kff.org

Long Term Care Provider.com: http://www.longtermcareprovider.com

Mayo Clinic: http://www.mayoclinic.com

Medscape: http://www.medscape.com

Modern Healthcare: http://www.modernhealthcare.com

MultiMedia HealthCare (MMHC): http://www.mmhc.com

National Alliance for Caregiving: http://www.caregiving.org

National Alliance on Mental Illness (NAMI): http://www.nami.org

National Association for Home Care & Hospice: http://www.nahc.org

National Association of County and City Health Officials (NACCHO):
  http://www.naccho.org

National Center for Assisted Living (NCAL): http://www.ahcancal.org/ncal

National Committee for Quality Assurance (NCQA): http://www.ncqa.org

National Council on Aging (NCOA): http://www.ncoa.org

The Rand Corporation: http://www.rand.org

Utilization Review Accreditation Commission (URAC): http://www.urac.org

Policy and Politics Journals

- American Politics Journal
- Economic Analysis and Policy
- Environmental Politics
- Ethics and Global Politics
- Health Affairs
- International Journal of E-Politics
- International Journal of Politics, Culture, and Society
- The International Journal of Sociology and Social Policy
- Journal of Economic Policy Reform
- Journal of Gender Law and Policy
- Journal of Health Politics, Policy, and Law
- Journal of Health Care Law and Policy
- Journal of Health Politics
- Journal of Health Services Research and Policy
- Journal of Information Technology and Politics
- Journal of International Aging, Law, and Policy
- Journal of Law and Politics
- Journal of Law, Economics, and Policy
- Journal of Legislation and Public Policy
- Journal of Mental Health Policy and Economics

- *Journal of Political Science, Government, and Politics*
- *Journal of Policy Analysis and Management*
- *Journal of Policy History*
- *Journal of Politics*
- *Journal of Politics and Law*
- *Journal of Public Health Policy*
- *Journal of Public Policy and Marketing*
- *Muckraker: Journal of the Center for Investigative Reporting*
- *Policy, Politics, and Nursing Practice*
- *Policy Studies Journal*
- *Political Science and Politics*
- *Politics and Society*
- *Public Citizen*
- *Whittier Law Review*
- *World Policy Journal*
- *World Politics*

INDEX

Pages followed by t or f denote tables or figures respectively.